Callanetics

am/pm
Callanetics

Callan Pinckney

ARROW

Published in 1993 by Vermilion Arrow
an imprint of Ebury Press
Random House UK Ltd
20 Vauxhall Bridge Road
London SW1V 2SA

3 5 7 9 10 8 6 4 2

A catalogue record for this book is available from the
British Library

Typeset in Concorde and Futura

Designed by Roger Walker
Photography by Stuart M. Gross

ISBN 0 09 922991 9

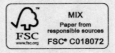

MIX
Paper from
responsible sources
FSC® C018072

Printed and bound in Great Britain by Clays Ltd, St Ives plc

For information on CALLANETICS® Studio Franchises or CALLANETICS® classes: contact

Callanetics Franchising Corp.,
1600 Stout Street, Suite 555, Denver,
Colorado 80202. (303) 572-7517.

WARNING:

There are risks inherent in any exercise programme. The advice of a doctor should be obtained prior to embarking on any exercise regimen. This programme is intended for persons in good health.

TO PREGNANT WOMEN:

Under no circumstances should any woman in the first three months of pregnancy do any of the exercises featured in this book which also use the stomach muscles. After the first three months do not attempt to do these exercises unless your doctor has actually done them to feel how deep the contractions are. These exercises appear to be very easy, but looks in this case are extremely deceiving.

Contents

Introduction

Welcome to *am/pm Callanetics*, a complete exercise programme that works on your entire body and is designed to get you into your best possible shape – quickly and safely.

We live in a hectic, stressful world. I know how busy most of you are and how important it is for you to get the most out of the time you spend exercising, so I have devised *am/pm Callanetics* to meet those needs. Its unique format features two complete, highly effective morning and evening workouts that not only improve your body shape but also improve your energy levels and reduce stress.

This entire am/pm programme takes only forty minutes – twenty minutes in the morning, and twenty minutes in the evening. By breaking up the time you spend exercising in this way, you should find it easier to fit this programme into your daily schedule and you will see results faster. The morning programme will give you renewed vitality so that you have greater strength, aliveness and energy to start your day, while the evening programme will completely relax you, enabling you to shed the tensions of the day, leave its stresses behind, and allowing you to have a peaceful night's sleep. And, of course, the wonderful bonus is that you will have a terrific body twenty-four hours a day!

Like all Callanetics programmes, these am/pm routines work deeply on *all* your muscles and you'll see extremely fast results. Your body will quickly become tight, shapely and beautiful, your posture will improve, and you will be ecstatic at the new burst of energy you will experience. If you are dieting, it will often look as if you have lost twice the weight, because Callanetics pulls your muscles up and in so effectively.

Callanetics strengthens, without impact. The exercises are designed to protect your back, as well as every other part of your body. In no time at all you will look and feel truly amazing. Whatever your age or ability, you will soon find that your muscles are able to do things that seemed impossible the last time you tried. And it's simple to learn.

A Positive Self-Image

By practising this programme regularly, not only will you notice a wonderful transformation of your figure, but as you learn to be in control of your body you will also feel more alert, your self-confidence will increase and you will be motivated to do so much more in your life. And feeling in control of your body actually helps to reduce stress. My goal is to help you to develop a positive attitude – towards your body and your life.

Nina, who demonstrates the exercises in this book, is a living example of what Callanetics can do for you. Nina is thirty-eight years old with three children, all delivered by Caesarean section. She first started to practise Callanetics in 1987. Years of practising high-impact aerobics had caused her countless injuries over the years. In particular, she suffered extreme pain in her lower back and constant pinches in her neck and shoulders. At one point she was in such considerable pain that she was unable even to turn her head. Endless courses of drugs and medication offered little in the way of permanent relief. However, since she started to practise Callanetics she has undergone a miraculous transformation. Performing the small, gentle movements of Callanetics and learning how to relax her body has left her completely free of pain, and she has suffered no further injuries. At the same time, her body became tighter, stronger and more shapely – the results were phenomenal. Just look at the photographs, and you will see what I mean.

Nina was so delighted with the results that she wanted to share her knowledge and use her experience to enthuse others. She therefore underwent intense training as a Callanetics teacher and subsequently acquired her own Callanetics franchise. Two years ago, she set up her own studio in Potomac, Maryland, just outside Washington DC. Nina feels very excited and positive about her life, since not only is she contributing to her own well-being, she is also able to contribute to the well-being of others by offering practical support, encouragement and motivation.

So What Is Callanetics and How Does It Work?

Callanetics is a series of stretching and contracting exercises that activate the body's largest muscle groups, using tiny, gentle, precise movements, called pulses. They are done very slowly in what I call 'triple slow motion', reaching deep into the muscles to give you a strong, firm body, without adding bulk.

I first devised my original Callanetics programme in an attempt to avoid surgery on my back and my knees. I have a long history of back problems, since I was born with curvature of the spine, and after leaving college eleven years of backpacking around the world and undertaking a variety of hard manual labouring jobs to make ends meet also took its toll. My back and knees deteriorated further, and, on returning to the United States, I was determined to do something about my pitiful physical condition. However, I found that the exercises in the classes I attended put a huge strain on my back. I therefore experimented with other techniques, incorporating movements learned while studying classical ballet as a child, and gradually evolved a way of shifting my body position and moving in a slow, gentle way that protected my back. In addition to correcting my physical problems, I was amazed to see how strong and tight my body had become. My posture improved, and I looked and felt years youngers. Friends begged me to let them in on my secret, and that

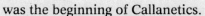

was the beginning of Callanetics.

Think of Callanetics as meditation in motion. You reach into the body to work the large muscle groups, as though working through them layer by layer, using movements as small and delicate as a pulse. There are no jerking or bouncing movements in Callanetics. Callanetics is and always has been no-impact. Some people have even called it the 'no effort' exercise, but as anyone who has experienced Callanetics will tell you it only looks effortless. It is not difficult to do, but you will feel your muscles working, as these tiny movements are in fact incredibly powerful, providing an extremely fast, safe and effective way of achieving a strong, more youthful-looking body.

I like to say that Callanetics defies gravity, because every second of every day gravity is pulling your muscles down, causing your body to droop, sag and spread over the years. With Callanetics, however, as you work to get your muscles strong, your muscles will lift, taking the skin with them and restoring everything to a more youthful position, producing those sleek, tight body contours we all so admire.

In all the exercises the emphasis is on techniques that prevent you from putting any strain on the lower back. By stretching the spine at the same time you are working the surrounding muscles, pressure on your back will be alleviated, and stretching the spine will also improve your posture. As the neck region and the area between the shoulder blades loosen, it becomes easier to pull your shoulders back and stand more erect. The neck appears longer, and this can have the effect of making you appear taller. Whatever your shape or size, Callanetics can enhance your appearance by tightening your muscles more than you ever dreamed possible. And it takes only a few hours to see truly astounding results.

In short, Callanetics produces the fastest results in the shortest possible time – with no injuries. At the same time it protects and strengthens your back. The tiny, precise, delicate pulsing movements will also work your heart in a very gentle way. Whatever your age, sex or physical condition, it's not too late to rejuvenate your body and achieve a fantastic figure. You can have the beautiful, powerful body you deserve, if you're willing to work for it.

How to Get the Most Out of This Programme

The daily routines in *am/pm Callanetics* form a complete and balanced programme of carefully constructed stretching and contracting exercises that work on the entire body and rejuvenate the major muscle groups. Your muscles will be gently stretched and your joints delicately put through their whole range of movement to protect your body from injury.

It is up to you how many times a week you practise this programme, but try to do it at least three times a week. The more often you practise

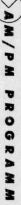

the programme, the faster you will see results. It is perfectly safe to do every day, if you wish, since these exercises, with their delicate, controlled movements, do not cause the wear and tear that weights, jerking and the impact movements often used in other forms of exercise involve. You will be working your muscles at your own pace, without fear of exhaustion or injury, and your muscles will work only at the level at which they are capable of performing, without forcing. To get the maximum benefits from this programme, always try to do both the am and pm routines on the days that you exercise. If you are pushed for time, you can split the programme so that you practise the am and pm routines on alternate days – whatever works for you time-wise – but your body will respond better to the exercises and you will shape up more quickly if you do both routines on the same day.

Before You Start

Before attempting each exercise, make sure you have read all the instructions so that you have a clear idea of how to proceed. Remember that many of the photographs show the ultimate position that can be achieved for each exercise, so do not expect to attain these positions immediately. Just be patient, and eventually you will be amazed at how much you are capable of stretching and strengthening your body.

Most of the exercises give instructions for both easier and more advanced alternatives so that you

are able to work at your own level and progress at your own pace. If you are not able to do the 'standard' version of a particular exercise, start off slowly with the easier option and build yourself up gradually before progressing to the more advanced alternatives. Once you have learned the correct position for a given exercise you will find you progress more quickly and the exercises will soon become second nature. As you become more familiar with the routines and you learn how to relax your entire body, you'll soon find these exercises become the highlight of your day. You don't need any special clothing or equipment. You can do them on a mat in your bedroom, even watching your favourite television programme, using a piece of furniture for balance. Try to make these exercises part of your everyday life.

Always do the routines in the exact sequence as outlined in the book. Start with the warm-ups, then proceed with the exercises and stretches in the order they are given. It is important to work the muscles in a certain sequence so that they do not become fatigued. Each exercise is designed to complement the one that follows. The stretches will also stretch the specific muscles you have been working to help prevent injury and to lengthen the muscles after they have been contracted to prevent them from developing bulk.

Total relaxation

Throughout this book you will find I ask you over and over again to relax your body while doing an exercise. Relaxation is one of the first things I teach my students, since people who have not experienced Callanetics before find it difficult to understand how they can relax while working a muscle. All I am asking you to do is not to forcefully tense your muscles, since any more contracting or stretching than is necessary to perform the required movement creates extra work for your muscles and wastes valuable energy. It also prevents you from reaching the level you are capable of achieving. Relaxing your body allows the muscles to work more deeply. It also takes the pressure off your lower back and protects you from injury. By training yourself to relax while working a muscle, whether stretching or contracting, you will be in control of the motion rather than it taking control of you.

Use your exercise time as an opportunity to calm your thoughts. Just relax, and think beautiful, soft, gentle thoughts. Feel your entire body from the top of your head to your toes become like wax melting into the floor. Exert the minimum amount of effort for the maximum results. The more you relax, the more you will find you are able to do, because you will not be exhausting the muscles, and the faster the exercises will work.

Triple slow motion

Because it is so important that you control the motion, rather than letting the motion control you, throughout this book I ask you to move *in triple slow motion*. Imagine you are watching a slow-

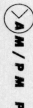

motion sequence in a film or television programme. Now slow the movement down even
more. This is triple slow motion. The only excep-
tions to this rule are the warm-up exercises Up and
Down (am programme) and The Swing (pm programme), where you should move in *slow motion*.

All your movements should be gentle, flowing
and delicate. Never jerk or bounce, but treat your
body with the respect it deserves.

No forcing

Do not under any circumstances force your body
to do anything it is not prepared to do. Pushing the
body to do too much too soon or forcing the muscles beyond their limitations can result in exhaustion of injury. Never stretch more than you are
capable of stretching. Your muscles will stretch in
their own time. Every stretch should feel comfortable; never do it to the point of pain. By not forcing, you will gain the full benefit of an exercise. Let
gentleness control the motion.

Always work at your own pace

Don't be discouraged if you are not able to do the
specified number of repetitions of an exercise
when you first start. This is natural because you
will probably be using muscles you have never
used in your entire life before. You must give them
a chance to build up strength. If an instruction
asks for 100 pulses and you can only do 20 at first,
then that is your level. Just do what you can. You

won't see results as quickly, but your safety comes first. Always listen to your body. It will let you know when it is ready to do more. As you become stronger, you will be able to increase the number of repetitions with ease and you'll be up to 100 in no time.

Don't expect your body to respond to exercise in the same way each day, and never compare your progress with another person's. Everyone's body is different, and some people's bodies have more flexibility than others'.

Take a breather whenever you feel in need of one. If you stop to take a breather, always make sure you resume the original starting position again before continuing the exercise, following the instructions step by step. Count your repetitions carefully and always be sure to do the same number to each side to ensure you are strengthening, tightening and pulling in both sides of your body equally.

Pain

When you use a muscle in a new way, or stretch one that has not been used before, it is normal to feel a slight sensation in the area being worked. If this happens, and it feels too uncomfortable, you can shift position or modify the movement to make yourself more comfortable as long as you are still working the muscle, or you can try working the opposite side or take a breather. Then when you resume the exercise, continue the count where you left off.

However, if you feel any sudden or sharp stabbing pain – especially in the chest or arm, which could indicate angina – breathlessness or dizziness, stop immediately. If the pain continues or worsens, you should consult a doctor as it could indicate a pre-existing medical condition.

Breathing

Some people concentrate on complicated breathing techniques they have been taught by other exercise instructors instead of concentrating on the exercises. This often results in tensing the body when it should be relaxed. For this reason, there are no special breathing instructions for Callanetics. Just breathe naturally – but do remember to breathe! Some people tend to hold their breath when exercising.

Counting

Several of the exercises include instructions for a specific number of pulses or to hold for a certain count. You should count 'one thousand and one, one thousand and two' etc. If you count aloud, an added plus is that you will be conscious of your breathing.

Equipment

Although there is no special equipment needed in order to practise this programme, some of the exercises call for the use of a barre. You can use almost any sturdy piece of furniture, such as a table, the back of a sofa or chair. Before you begin, make sure it is strong enough to support your weight, and choose a height that is comfortable for you. In the photographs in this book, Nina is using only a lightweight stool at a low height, since her body is strong and needs no support.

You may also need to use a mat or towel to cushion your back, knees or buttocks in the exercises performed on the floor.

It is advisable not to wear shoes for any of these exercises. The weight of them is simply too heavy and they throw you off your natural balance. Under no circumstances should you place weights on your arms or legs.

Music

If you wish to exercise to music, make sure that it is soft and soothing so that you feel calm, relaxed and able to concentrate. Never play hard jerky music, as you will tend to try to keep up with the beat and this can encourage bouncing and jerking motions and force you to lose control.

And remember ...

Each time you exercise, think of the key words and phrases in Callanetics:

Relax your entire body
Your body is like a rag doll
Let your body melt into the floor

Think beautiful, soft, gentle thoughts
Always move in *triple slow motion*
Let gentleness control the motion
Always work at your own pace
Listen to your body
Never force the movement
Never stretch more than you are capable of
   stretching
Your muscles will stretch when they are ready to
   stretch, not when you command them
Never jerk or bounce
Do not force
Your movements should be almost imperceptible
   – gentle and delicate, like a pulse
When pulsing, never move more than $1/4$ to $1/2$
   inch
Take a breather whenever you feel in need of one

Curling Up the Pelvis

If there is one movement that is key to Callanetics,
it is curling up the pelvis, the link between the
upper and lower body. The pelvic area is possibly
the most important structure affecting the posture,
balance and alignment of the body, especially in
everyday life, and is crucial for supporting your
entire back. By learning how to allow the pelvic
area to function in the way it was created to, you
will experience feelings of freedom and release and
derive benefits for the entire body. There are no
muscles used solely for moving the pelvis, but the
muscles of the legs and torso control its move-

ment. The pelvic curl-up can be done lying down, standing or sitting. When you first start to practise it, if you are standing, always bend your knees so that you can really feel how your pelvis is curling up. As your body becomes stronger and you become more familiar with this movement, you will experience no difficulty in curling your pelvis up and in certain exercises you will be able to keep your legs straight with your knees relaxed.

To do the pelvic curl-up, tighten your buttocks and, *in triple slow motion*, try to move or 'curl up'

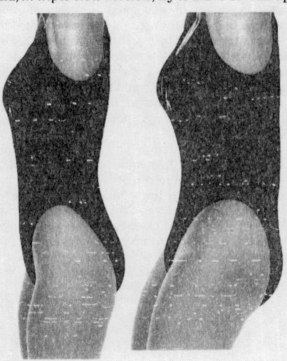

the pelvic area as if you were trying to get your pubic bone to curl up and in towards your navel. Imagine there is a string attached to the crotch of your leotard. Gently pull up on the string, and your pelvis will curl up. This movement strengthens your abdominal, inner- and front thigh, and buttock muscles, as well as loosening the hip joints and allowing for more fluid movements. If you are standing, it also strengthens your calves and feet.

Once you have perfected the curl, you will feel the lower back stretching and you will have much more flexibility in the spine. As your muscles become stronger, you will be able to increase the degree of the curl. The more the pelvis is curled up, the deeper the buttock muscles contract and the faster the results. Remember, you can always curl your pelvis up more than you think you can. When you are free of tension after doing the pelvic curl-up, your energy and your body will feel beautiful, light and flowing.

This is one exercise you can practise anywhere, any time. Remember, it does not mean sticking out your stomach or arching your back. It is a gentle rounding up, a graceful flowing movement. When your pelvis starts to have that beautiful flow, there will be no excuse for slumping over. You will be able to curl up your pelvis with ease as you walk, stand and sit. This will allow you to stretch your spine more comfortably to its limit and hold your head and shoulders erect.

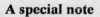

A special note

With all exercises that require you to curl up the pelvis, the more you tighten your buttocks and curl your pelvis up, the more you will protect your back. If you have a swayback, always curl your pelvis up as much as you possibly can.

This **am programme** will get your day off to a perfect start. As you perform these exercises, prepare your mind and body to meet this new day and all of its challenges with greater strength, energy and a positive self-image. Feel your muscles relax and become stronger, while your energy level reaches new heights.

The am Programme

WARM-UPS

Up and Down

Feel 2 inches taller!

> This exercise:
> - stretches the spine
> - loosens the knees

This entire exercise should be performed in one *slow*, *smooth*, continuous motion.

▶ Stand with your feet a hip-width apart and your knees slightly bent. Stretch both arms up to the ceiling as high as you can, at the same time stretching your torso up. Tighten your buttocks and curl your pelvis up (see page 22). Now, stretch your torso up even more. Keep your knees relaxed; don't lock them.

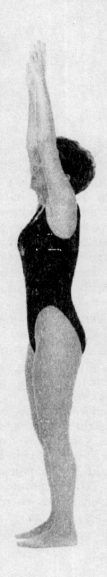

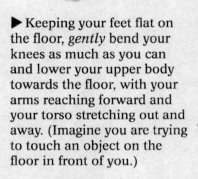

▶ Keeping your feet flat on the floor, *gently* bend your knees as much as you can and lower your upper body towards the floor, with your arms reaching forward and your torso stretching out and away. (Imagine you are trying to touch an object on the floor in front of you.)

▶ *Very gently* swing your arms back, raising them as high as you can behind your body, and at the same time totally relax your neck. Your knees will straighten slightly and your buttocks will rise with the motion of your arms going to the back of you and then up. (This position is one of the few instances where your pelvis is not curled up.)

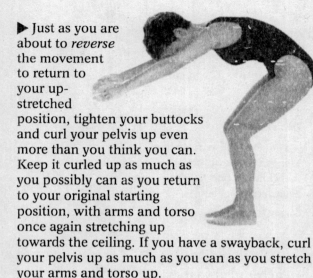

▶ Just as you are about to *reverse* the movement to return to your up-stretched position, tighten your buttocks and curl your pelvis up even more than you think you can. Keep it curled up as much as you possibly can as you return to your original starting position, with arms and torso once again stretching up towards the ceiling. If you have a swayback, curl your pelvis up as much as you can as you stretch your arms and torso up.

REPETITIONS
 5

REMEMBER

- When stretching your arms and torso up towards the ceiling keep your pelvis curled up as much as you possibly can; do not arch your back.

- Do not lock your knees or tense your feet.

- Relax your shoulders and neck; don't tense them.

AM PROGRAMME

The Waist Stretch

An alternative to wearing
corsets!

This exercise:

- stretches the waist, hips,
  spine, back of the
  shoulders and the
  underarm area
- reduces the waist

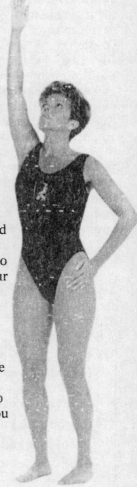

▶ Stand with your feet a hip-
width apart. Put your left hand
on or just below your left hip,
with your elbow out directly to
the side. This is to protect your
lower back. Reach your right
arm up as high as you can,
your palm facing inwards.
Bend your knees slightly.
*Tighten your buttocks and
curl your pelvis up* even more
than you think you can to
protect your back. Now, try to
reach up even higher, until you
feel your leotard or clothing
moving up your right side.
This will stretch your torso
and waist even more.

▶ Keeping your right arm stretched and as straight as possible, and with your pelvis still curled up, gently lean directly over to your left side as far as you can, without forcing. *In triple slow motion*, pulse your torso (not your arm) up and down, no more than 1/4 to 1/2 inch, while stretching your torso over to the left in a smooth, continuous motion. Make sure your neck and your left shoulder are relaxed.

▶ To come out of this stretch, instead of standing up straight (as this would put pressure on your lower back), *gently* bend your knees *as much as you can* and continue to stretch your right arm over to your left side. In one smooth, continuous motion bring your right arm and torso around to the front of you, *slowly* extending them down towards the floor and then over to your right side. Feel your spine stretching.

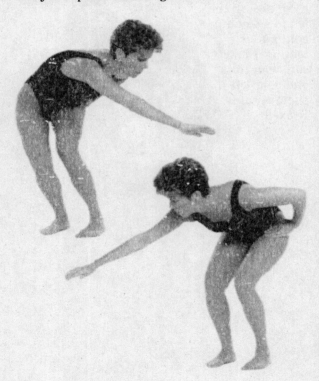

▶ When you feel that your back is totally relaxed and that you can't go any further to the right, slowly come up to your original starting position by tightening your buttocks, *curling up your pelvis* and rounding up your torso vertebra by vertebra. Gently lift your head up last of all.

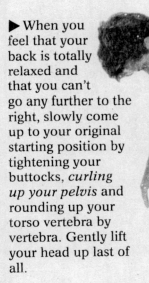

REPETITIONS
to each side

▶▶ Start with 75 pulses

▶▶ Work up to 100 pulses

Note: *When you become more stretched, you will experience no difficulty in curling up your pelvis. When this happens you will be able to keep your knees straight without locking them.*

35

IF YOU FEEL PRESSURE ON YOUR LOWER BACK:

As you lean over to your left side, bend your knees even more and bring your right arm and torso forward, so that your right arm is reaching out diagonally across your body, or out at shoulder height (whichever is more comfortable), and your right hand is in line with your left shoulder.

REMEMBER

- You can always stretch over more than you think you can.

- Relax your head, shoulders and neck.

- Do not tense your legs or feet.

- Keep your knees relaxed; don't lock them.

- Do not stick your buttocks out or push your stomach forward.

- Keep your outstretched arm as straight as you can and as close to your head as possible.

- Relax the shoulder of the arm that is resting on your hip.

- Do not bounce up and down. Your pulses should be almost imperceptible.

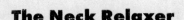
The Neck Relaxer

Relaxation – plain and simple.

> **This exercise:**
> - loosens the neck and shoulders
> - stretches the spine
> - keeps the neck area flexible

Note: *Always move in triple slow motion and think beautiful, soft, gentle thoughts.*

▶ Stand erect with your feet a hip-width apart, knees slightly bent. Relax your shoulders – feel as if they are melting into the floor – and relax your arms. Stretch the back of the neck up and look straight ahead. (Imagine there is a string running from the top your head to the ceiling, pulling your head up and stretching your neck even more.) Relax your jaw.

▶ *In triple slow motion*, turn your head as if trying to look over your right shoulder to have a conversation with someone standing behind you. Keep both shoulders relaxed and facing the front – don't rotate them. Very gently and slowly, turn your head to the front again.

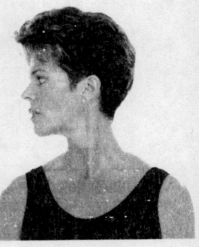

▶ Then, *still slowly*, turn your head to where you are looking over your left shoulder. Finally, slowly move your head back to the centre. A movement to both sides counts as one repetition.

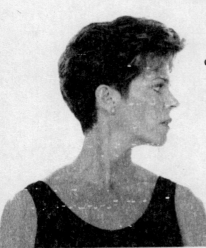

REPETITIONS
to each side
▶▶ 3

REMEMBER

- Keep your shoulders relaxed, as if they were melting into the floor. Don't let them move up – as they tend to do naturally when you are stretching your neck up, if you're not thinking about it.

- As you move your head, do not turn your body or rotate your shoulders.

- Do not jerk your neck as you move it.

- Do not stick out your buttocks or your stomach. Keep your buttocks tightened and your pelvis curled up.

- Do not tense your feet or lock your knees.

Note: *As your muscles relax even more, you will be able to curl up your pelvis more to stretch your spine, and you won't have to bend your knees as much.*

LEGS AND INNER THIGHS

You will need a barre for the following exercise. You can use almost any sturdy piece of furniture such as a table, the back of a sofa or chair. Before you begin, make sure it is robust enough to support your weight, and choose a height that is comfortable for you. Nina is using only a lightweight stool, since her body is extremely strong and needs no support. The height of this stool will probably be too low for most people at first. When you become stronger you can vary the height as you wish. However, unless you are very tall, your barre should never be higher than 56 inches.

At first your torso may be rounded towards the barre and you will be holding on to the barre for dear life. As you become stronger, you will eventually be able to hold your torso perfectly erect, and your hands will simply be resting on the barre.

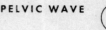

The Pelvic Wave

The way to leaner, longer-looking legs.

This exercise:

- strengthens and tightens the legs, the buttocks and the abdominal muscles

- works the front and inner thighs, feet, ankles and calves

- stretches the spine and the area between the shoulder blades

- keeps the pelvis flexible for health purposes

Note: If you have knee problems or weak knees, do this exercise very gently and slowly. Placing the heels together helps to distribute and stabilize the body's weight more effectively and takes pressure off the knees. If this doesn't help at first, you can place your feet flat on the floor, a hip-width apart, toes facing forward. I have received many letters from people who have found this exercise has helped to alleviate knee problems due to injuries, arthritis, or even surgery, and many of my students have reported that it improved their condition tremendously. You'll find that practising this exercise can actually help decrease the likelihood of further injuries in other activities, by strengthening your leg muscles. Since these muscles are the

*same ones that assist the back muscles in
everyday activities, the extra bonus is you'll be
less likely to have problems running, walking or
standing. Just be gentle with yourself, and if
you do not feel confident, go on to
the next exercise and return to
this one when your body
becomes stronger.*

▶ Stand facing and holding on to
your barre or piece of furniture,
with your feet turned out to the
sides. Go up on to the balls of your
feet, heels together, knees bent and
arms straight but relaxed. Do not
arch your back – keep it straight
and relaxed, if possible – and do
not force the knees out to the
sides at all.
Now, *in triple
slow motion,*
with your torso

erect but relaxed, if possible, and your neck relaxed and stretching towards the ceiling, lower your torso 2 inches straight down towards the floor, keeping your heels together.

▶ Tighten your buttocks and curl your pelvis up, aiming it up and in towards your navel. Then curl your pelvis up even more than you think you can, and at the same time allow your upper torso to round as much as possible. Gently release your pelvis without pushing your buttocks back, allowing your torso to move back to the centre.

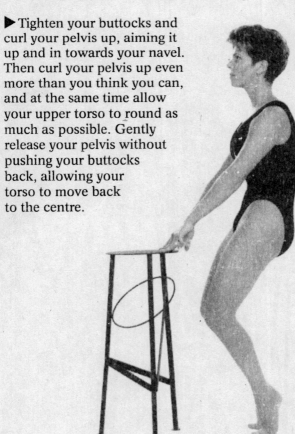

▶ *In triple slow motion*, go down 2 more inches, tighten your buttocks, curl your pelvis up even more, and gently release.

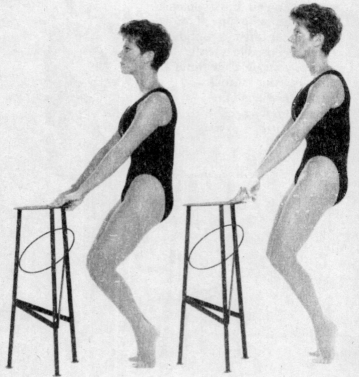

▶Go down another 2 inches, tighten your buttocks, curl your pelvis up even more, and gently release. Feel how much your inner thighs are working at this level.

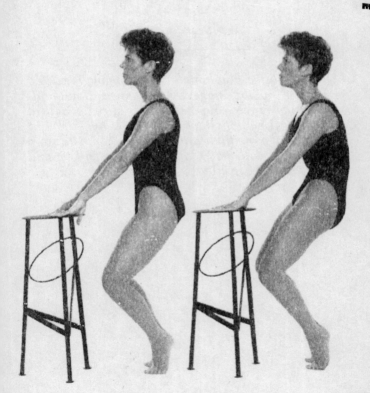

▶ Now reverse the movement, going up 2 inches, tightening your buttocks, curling your pelvis up and then releasing each time, just as slowly, until you have returned to your original standing position. This entire sequence counts as one repetition.

> **REPETITIONS**
> ▶▶ Start with 3
> ▶▶ Work up to 5

Note: Notice how much Nina's pelvis is curled up (see previous page). At first you will not realize how much your pelvis can curl up with a beautiful, smooth flow. You can always curl your pelvis up more than you think you can. The more you relax your body, the easier this will be and the faster the results.

REMEMBER

- For the second and third repetitions, you should curl your pelvis up even more each time.

- When coming out of the pelvic curl, do not stick your buttocks out or arch your back. Your spine is always straight when your pelvis is not curled up.

- Let the position of the knees be natural; do not aim them too far out to the sides.

- Keep your shoulders relaxed.

- For the most beneficial spine stretch, your upper back should be as rounded as possible when curling up the pelvis. The more your pelvis is curled up, the more your torso will round, stretching the spine, and the faster your legs will become strong and tight.

- When your legs become strong, train yourself not to lean your weight on the barre. Keep your balance on the balls of your feet.

- When lowering your torso, do not allow your buttocks to drop below your knees. This puts too much pressure on your knees.

COMING UP OFF THE FLOOR

Before moving on to the stomach exercises, take a minute or two to practise coming up off the floor without putting pressure on your back.

One of the worst things you can do for your back is to jerk yourself up off the floor and just get up. It is simple to learn how to get up gracefully in a fluid, easy motion. Always follow these directions after doing exercises or stretches on the floor.

▶ Lying on your back on the floor with your knees bent and relaxed, your feet a hip-width apart and flat on the floor, gently roll your bent knees, one at a time, over to the right, and then roll your torso over to the right. Now, keeping your knees on the floor, place your left palm on the floor to the right of you. Using the strength of your left hand, and supporting your weight on your right arm, *in triple slow motion* start lifting your body up. Then place your right palm on the floor and, walking your hands on the floor, gently ease yourself up until you are sitting on your heels.

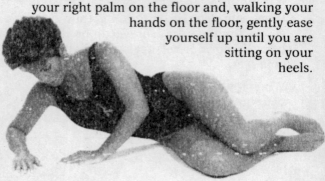

▶*In triple slow motion*, take your left leg up, bent, to where your left foot is resting on the floor. Do not lock your elbows.

▶ Bring your right leg up. Then tighten your buttocks and curl your pelvis up.

▶ Now, keeping your head down, *in triple slow motion* gently straighten up one vertebra at a time until you are in a standing position. Gently lift your head up last of all.

49

STOMACH

The next two stomach exercises:

• tighten the abdominal muscles from the breastbone to the pubis
• release the tension in the back of the neck
• lengthen the neck
• release the tension across the shoulder blades
• increase breathing capacity by expanding the chest
• lift the breasts by strengthening the pectoral muscles
• protect the back
• release tension in, stretch and increase the flexibility of, the entire back
• reduce double chins
• assist in regulating bowel movements
• help to control the appetite (for most people)
• help lessen monthly discomfort for women

At first glance, these exercises may look like many other stomach exercises, but let me explain why they are very different indeed. This may seem like a lot of information to absorb at first, but once your body starts to respond to the directions, this will all become second nature to you, and you will be astounded at the incredible results these exercises can produce.

The stomach exercises in this programme are not traditional sit-ups. A traditional sit-up requires you to thrust your entire upper body up off the floor, thereby creating a terrific struggle against gravity and pushing the stomach muscles far beyond their capacity. Other muscle groups, particularly the back muscles, are therefore brought in to assist the stomach muscles, putting excessive pressure on the lower back. However, with Callanetics the body is positioned in a particular way so that you learn to relax your entire body and place no strain whatsoever on your stomach or back muscles. Your stomach muscles will then automatically work at the level at which they are capable of performing, without forcing. Since the stomach muscles will be working in isolation, without the assistance of other muscle groups, you will do fewer repetitions at first than you would of a traditional sit-up. However, since you will be working the stomach muscles more deeply, the benefits will be much greater. When your muscles become stronger at this deeper level, you will be able to increase the number of repetitions.

Do these exercises very slowly and gently, letting your lower back melt into the floor and without tensing your stomach or buttock muscles. *And remember, as you do your tiny pulsing movements, your head, arms and upper torso move together as a unit*. Many beginners make the mistake of moving just one body part, either the neck, or the arms or the upper torso.

At first you will feel the muscles contracting just below the chest. As your muscles become stronger in that area, the contractions will be felt lower down. This process continues until you are working the muscles just above the pubic bone. As your abdominals begin to pull in, the lower abdomen may appear to protrude. Don't panic (as I did). Unless you have an allergy or digestive problem that is causing bloat and needs medical attention, your stomach will flatten as the lower abdominals catch up. If you do not see visible results after the first six sessions and your stomach appears puffy or swollen, it is possible you may have a pre-existing medical disorder, and you should consult your doctor.

Note: Some people may feel a slight discomfort in the back of their neck the first few times they attempt these exercises. This is natural at first, since the neck is where many people hold tension from the stress of everyday living, and it is this tension that creates the discomfort. Learning to relax as you do these exercises will help to loosen the neck muscles and release the tension, as well as producing faster results. Should you find it too uncomfortable, you can clasp your hands behind your head and let your head rest in the palms of your hands, keeping your elbows out to the sides, as you perform the movements. The discomfort should disappear after the first few sessions. You will then experience a sensation in the muscles at both sides of the neck. Be grateful for this lat-ter sensation as these are the muscles which make the neck look longer. However, if the dis-comfort in the back of the neck persists, you should consult a doctor as this could be a signal of a pre-existing chronic disc problem.

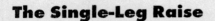

The Single-Leg Raise

The fastest way to a flat tummy.

Note: Most people don't realize that they can actually point their toes without tensing their leg muscles. In the following exercises, whenever one leg or both legs are raised, point your toes but remember to keep your feet and legs perfectly relaxed. This is a wonderful opportunity to start training yourself to relax different parts of your body.

▶ Lie on the floor with your knees bent and aiming up towards the ceiling, feet a hip-width apart and flat on the floor. Bend your right knee in towards your chest as far as you can.

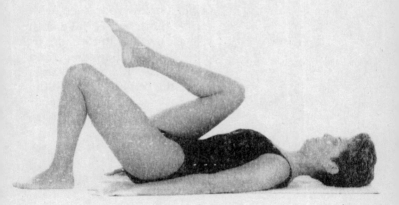

53

▶ *Gently* raise your right leg straight up, with toes relaxed and pointing towards the ceiling. If you can't raise your leg straight up or straighten it at first, that's perfectly all right. In the beginning, just work at the level that feels comfortable for you.

▶ Now, *keeping your head on the floor*, grasp the back of your right thigh, just below your knee, with both hands. Take both elbows out to the sides as far as they can go and then aim them up towards the ceiling to stretch the area between your shoulder blades.

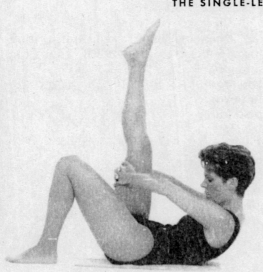

▶ Now, *in triple slow motion*, round your head and shoulders off the floor, bringing your head up first and aiming your nose and shoulders in towards your chest. At the same time, take your elbows out and then up even more to stretch the upper back. Always round your head and shoulders more than you think you can. Your middle- and lower back remain on the floor. Now, try to aim your nose in towards your chest even more.

▶ When you feel that you can't round any further in towards your chest, slowly straighten your left leg in front of you, raised no more than a foot off the floor. If that is too difficult at first, either rest your left leg on the floor or return your left leg to its starting position with the knee bent. Now, take your hands off your legs and place your arms by your sides, extending them straight out in front, palms down, 6 inches to 1 foot off the floor. From this position, *in triple slow motion* gently pulse your upper torso (not just your arms or head, or your entire torso) ¼ to ½ inch forward and back, allowing your entire body to melt into the floor.

▶ To come out of this exercise, *in triple slow motion* gently bend first your right knee and then your left knee so that both feet are resting on the floor, and slowly lower your head and shoulders back to the floor, rolling down vertebra by vertebra.

▶ Repeat this exercise on the opposite side.

> **REPETITIONS**
> to each side
> ▶▶ Start with 75 pulses
> ▶▶ Work up to 100 pulses

IF YOU NEED TO TAKE A BREATHER:

Grasp your right leg just below the knee with both hands, hold your rounded position with your elbows out, and breathe deeply and naturally. If you need to, bend your left knee and

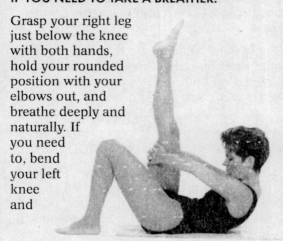

rest your left foot flat on the floor. To continue the count, return your left leg to its straightened position, and then take your elbows out and up even more before releasing your hands.

Or, if you prefer, you can bend first your right knee and then your left knee in towards your chest, then place both feet flat on the floor and gently lower your head and shoulders back to the floor, rolling down vertebra by vertebra. When you are ready to continue, follow the instructions step by step to return to your original position – that is, with the right leg straight up, foot relaxed and toes pointed towards the ceiling.

IF THIS EXERCISE IS TOO DIFFICULT AT FIRST, OR IF YOU FEEL PRESSURE ON YOUR LOWER BACK:

Gently bend your upstretched leg, or lower your head and shoulders back towards the floor, or do both, until the pressure on your back eases.

WHEN THIS EXERCISE BECOMES TOO EASY:

Start to lower your upstretched leg $1/2$ inch at a time. The lower your upstretched leg goes down to the floor, the more your stomach muscles will have to work, but they must be ready for such an intense workout.

If you feel your lower back starting to take over – which is a sign that your stomach muscles are not strong enough to work at that more difficult level – slowly raise your right leg back up towards the ceiling, $1/2$ inch at a time, until you feel no strain on your lower back.

Note: As soon as you release your hands to start your pulses, your shoulders will automatically tend to sink back down towards the floor. This is natural at first. When your muscles become stronger you will be able to keep your head and shoulders rounded and off the floor. The stronger your stomach muscles, the more you will be able to round your head and shoulders.

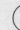

REMEMBER

- While getting into position keep your elbows aimed out to the sides and as high as you possibly can.

- When you are in the starting position, do not pull your leg to meet your face. Always make sure your leg is pointing towards the ceiling. As you become stronger, the leg may be lowered towards the floor.

- Keep your back relaxed; don't let it take over. How much you can round your upper back depends on how stretched your upper back muscles are, and how strong your stomach muscles have become.

- Try not to let your shoulders sink back down to the floor (as they will tend to do the first few times). Keep them rounded as much as you can. The more you can round your shoulders, the deeper the stomach muscles will work, producing faster results.

- Keep your body entirely relaxed, like a rag doll.

- Do not lock your knees.

- Do not tense your legs, stomach muscles or neck.

- Do not tighten your buttocks.

continued ...

- Never aim your face towards the ceiling; this puts a strain on your neck. Always aim your nose in towards your chest.

- Take breathers whenever you need to.

If for any reason you stop and come up off the floor after this exercise, make sure you follow the instructions on pages 48-49 on how to get up off the floor gracefully without putting pressure on your back.

The Double-Leg Raise

Flat, flatter, flattest!

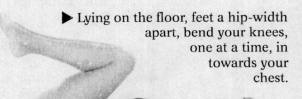

▶ Lying on the floor, feet a hip-width apart, bend your knees, one at a time, in towards your chest.

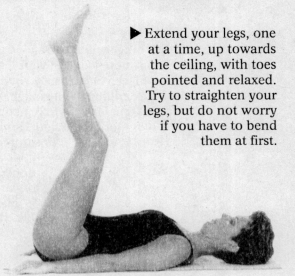

▶ Extend your legs, one at a time, up towards the ceiling, with toes pointed and relaxed. Try to straighten your legs, but do not worry if you have to bend them at first.

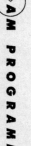

▶ Grasp your outer thighs with both hands, and aim your elbows out to the sides as much as you can and then up as high as you can. Gently round your head and shoulders off the floor even more than you think you can, aiming your nose and shoulders in towards your chest. At the same time, take your elbows out and up even more.

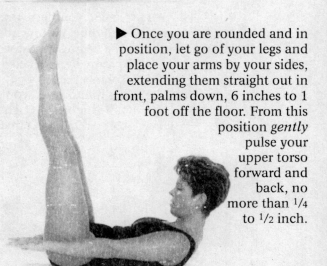

▶ Once you are rounded and in position, let go of your legs and place your arms by your sides, extending them straight out in front, palms down, 6 inches to 1 foot off the floor. From this position *gently* pulse your upper torso forward and back, no more than 1/4 to 1/2 inch.

▶ To come out of this exercise, *in triple slow motion* gently bend your knees and lower your feet to the floor, one at a time. Then slowly lower your head and shoulders back to the floor, rolling down vertebra by vertebra, totally relaxed.

REPETITIONS

▶▶ Start with 50 pulses

▶▶ Work up to 75 pulses

IF YOU NEED TO TAKE A BREATHER:

Grab hold of your outer thighs with both hands, hold your rounded position, with your elbows still aimed out to the sides, and breathe deeply and naturally.

Or you can bend both knees in towards your chest and roll back down to the floor, vertebra by vertebra. Before continuing the count, always make sure you return to your original starting position by taking your elbows out and up and rounding your head and shoulders in towards your chest.

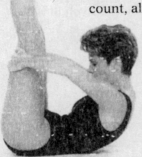

Note: At first, some people will do the exercise with knees bent. As you become stronger and more stretched, you will be able to round your head and shoulders more and straighten your legs with ease.

REMEMBER

- When you are getting into the starting position, aim your elbows out and up as far as they can go.

- Keep your head and shoulders rounded and off the floor as much as you can, aiming your nose in towards your chest.

- Try to relax your entire body, especially your legs and neck.

- Do not tense your buttocks or stomach muscles.

- Concentrate on letting your lower back melt into the floor.

- Take breathers whenever you need to.

Before beginning the next exercise you may need to come up off the floor to find a sturdy piece of furniture to use as a barre. Remember to reread the instructions on pages 48–49 on how to come up off the floor without putting pressure on your back.

BUTTOCKS, HIPS AND OUTER THIGHS

The next two exercises:

- resculpt the buttocks, giving them a 'precious peach' (instead of a 'sagging pear') shape
- round and lift the buttocks
- restore firmness
- get rid of the 'jiggle'
- reduce saddlebags, and eventually make them disappear
- strengthen the arm muscles

These exercises will counteract the effect of gravity that tugs at your bottom, causing it to droop, sag and spread over the years. Not only will you be working your buttock muscles to make your bottom tight and pulled up, so you achieve that fabulous round – like a peach – but at the same time you will be firming up your outer thighs and helping to banish that ugly outer thigh flab for ever! So you get two terrific benefits from each of these exercises.

When as a result of doing these exercises your bottom starts to pull up and in, you will experience a lump of flesh on both sides of your bottom about an inch below your waist. Don't worry. This is a signal that your buttock muscles are getting tighter and starting to pull the skin from your outer thighs round to your buttocks. As you continue to work the buttock muscles, they will become stronger and, in no time at all, they will lift up, taking the skin with them, and this area will smooth out to reshape your bottom to a childlike roundness.

The first few times you do these exercises you may feel a sensation in the hip of the working leg. If this happens, you can switch sides to work the other leg, and then return to the original side to continue the count where you left off. This sensation occurs because you are working the hip joints in a way they have not been worked for some time, or perhaps have never been worked at all. The joints weaken if they haven't been used and they haven't been doing what they were designed for. It's as if they have become rusty and need oiling. With Callanetics, however, you work the joints in the way that Nature intended, and the sensation you felt at first should soon disappear as the muscles become stronger.

Bringing Up the Rear (Sitting)

For a great rear view.

▶ Sit on your left buttock in front of your barre or piece of furniture, using a mat or towel to cushion yourself if necessary. Rest your left leg on the floor in front of you, with your left knee bent and aiming outwards and your left heel placed 8 to 10 inches away from the midline of your body. Your right leg is out to the side with its knee bent and the knee in line with your right hip. Your right foot rests on the floor behind you, with toes relaxed and aiming to the back of you. Both hips should be facing your barre.

▶ Place your left hand on your barre. Making sure that your right hip remains facing the barre, place your right hand on your right hip (*not* on your upper leg) to roll your right hip forward as much as you can.

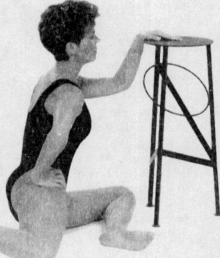

It will always roll forward more than you think it can. As your hip is rolled forward, your torso automatically turns to the left and your right foot should come off the floor. If it doesn't, use your right hand to assist it.

▶ Now, place your right hand on your barre and lift your right knee off the floor no more than 3 inches. Keep your right hip rolled forward and your torso straight and relaxed, if possible. *In triple slow motion*, pulse your knee backward, no more than 1/4 to 1/2 inch, and then forward so that your knee is

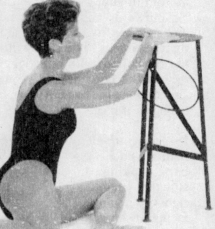

once again in line with your right hip. Try to relax your entire body, even though at first you will be holding on to the barre for dear life.

▶ Repeat this exercise on the opposite side.

REPETITIONS
to each side

▶▶ Start with 75 pulses

▶▶ Work up to 100 pulses

68

Note: At first it may seem impossible for you to lift your knee off the floor, much less pulse the knee ¹/₄ to ¹/₂ inch. If you find you are only able to do 5 pulses, just do 5 then take a breather. When you continue you will be surprised how many more pulses you are able to do. In no time at all, your muscles will become extremely strong and you will be able to roll your hip forward even more, causing your knee to be so low that it will almost seem to be brushing the floor. You will soon not need to use your hand to roll your hip forward and the exercise will seem like a breeze.

IF YOU FIND THE EXERCISE TOO DIFFICULT AT FIRST:

You can lean *directly* over to the opposite side of the leg you are working in order to be able to lift your knee off the floor.
You can also rest your hand on the floor to support your torso, or bring your working knee forward a little. Do not take your torso forward or push your stomach out, *(continued …)*

as that will cause you to arch your lower back, thereby putting pressure on it. In no time at all your muscles will become strong; your knee will be in line with your hip; you will be able to sit perfectly erect without support, and your pulsing leg will feel as light as a feather.

IF YOU FEEL IT'S TOO MUCH, AND YOUR BODY IS BEGINNING TO TENSE UP, OR IF YOU FEEL A SENSATION IN THE HIP OF THE WORKING LEG:

Take a breather, then roll your hip forward into position. You can also switch sides, but be sure to do a proper count for both sides. If you work one side more than the other you will end up with a lopsided bottom.

IF YOU FEEL PRESSURE ON YOUR LOWER BACK:

You have five options: you can round your upper back; lean over to the opposite side of your working leg just as much as you have to, keeping your back straight; place the opposite hand to the working knee on the floor to support your torso; bring your working knee forward a little; or, when nothing else works, tighten your buttocks and curl your pelvis up.

IF YOU WANT MORE OF A WORKOUT FOR YOUR BUTTOCKS:

Lower your foot a little bit, and then aim your kneecap towards the ceiling, but do not let your hip rotate to the back. For even more of a workout in this same position, you can also lift your knee and foot a wee bit more.

WHEN THIS EXERCISE BECOMES TOO EASY:

Be sure to sit more erect. You can also raise your barre, or place your hands higher up on your piece of furniture. The higher the barre, the more intense this exercise becomes. When your muscles become strong you may be able to sit erect and do the exercise without holding on to your barre at all.

Note: The more your hip is rolled forward, the more you will be working your buttock muscles. If you have a swayback, always round your upper back as much as you can. If your lower back arches as you roll your hip forward and you feel pressure on your lower back, you can let your torso lean over to the opposite side of the leg being used. This will stretch the spine even more and take the pressure off your lower back.

REMEMBER

- Do not arch your lower back.

- Do not push your stomach forward or out when rolling your hip forward. This will arch your lower back.

- Once you have lifted your knee off the floor and started your pulses, do not move your hip. Only the leg moves backward and forward.

- Keep your legs relaxed; don't tense them.

- Do not tense your neck.

- Do not hunch your shoulders.

- Your pulses should be barely perceptible.

- Do not allow the foot of your working leg to rest on the floor or your working knee to go forward. If your foot starts to feel heavy, take a breather.

- When rolling your hip forward do not allow your torso to push forward as this will put pressure on your lower back. Always keep your torso erect but relaxed, even if you are leaning your torso over to the side.

continued ...

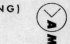

- When you become stronger, do not take the knee of your working leg past your hip when you are returning forward during the pulses.

- Keep your hips even.

- Work at your own pace. Relax into the floor and take a breather whenever you feel in need of one.

Out to the Side (Sitting)

For the tightest behind.

▶ Start in the same position as for the previous exercise, with your left leg bent and resting on the floor in front of you. Now, extend your right leg straight out to the side of your body so that your toes are even with your right hip, and place your left hand on your barre. Place your right hand on your right hip and slowly roll your right hip

and leg over so that the tops of your toes are trying to aim into the floor.

▶ Place your right hand on your barre and then pull your right leg in towards your body, letting your torso lean over directly to your left side if necessary.

▶ Now, lift your right foot off the floor no more than 3 inches and gently pulse it up and down, no more than $1/4$ to $1/2$ inch. (Do not take the leg to the back of you, as this is too advanced a workout for your muscles in the beginning.)

▶ Repeat on the opposite side.

REPETITIONS
to each side

▶▶ Start with 75 pulses

▶▶ Work up to 100 pulses

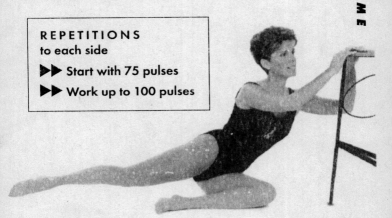

Notice how very little the foot is raised up off the floor. The movement can remain so small because the hip has been rolled forward so much.

Note: In the photographs above, you will notice that Nina is not sitting directly in front of the stool. In order for you to see clearly the position of the exercise, the angle of the stool has been adjusted for the purpose of these photographs.

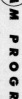

IF THIS EXERCISE IS TOO DIFFICULT AT FIRST:

Slowly ease your working leg forward a few inches, or bend your knee. You can also lean over further to the opposite side, or place the opposite hand to your working leg on the floor to the side of you. Take breathers whenever you have to.

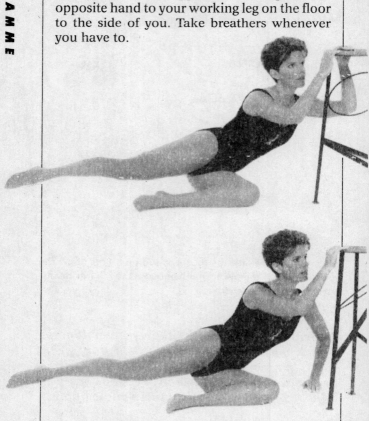

WHEN THIS EXERCISE BECOMES TOO EASY:

When your muscles are strong enough you can take your working leg to the back of you *without* rotating your hip back. You can also sit more erect, and roll your hip further forward. The more your hip is rolled forward, the more you will be working the buttock muscles.

IF YOU FEEL PRESSURE ON YOUR LOWER BACK:

Round your upper back, or lean over to the opposite side of your working leg just as much as you have to, keeping your back straight. You can also place your opposite hand on the floor to the side of you to support your torso. If nothing else works, tighten your buttocks and curl your pelvis up. If you have a sway-back, always round your upper back as much as you can to stop your back from arching. If that doesn't help, curl your pelvis up even more.

REMEMBER

- When rolling your hip forward, do not allow your torso or stomach to push forward as this will put pressure on your lower back. Keep your torso erect but relaxed, even if you are leaning over to the side.

- Always lift your leg from the foot, not the hip. Your hip should not move at all as you are doing your tiny pulses.

- Keep your extended leg very straight, but do not lock the knee.

- Keep your hips even.

- Keep your working hip forward as much as you can; don't let it roll back.

- Do not allow the foot of your working leg to rest on the floor. If your foot starts to feel heavy, take a breather.

- Never arch your back.

- Do not tense your neck.

- Do not hunch your shoulders.

- Totally relax your body, especially your shoulders.

- Work at your own pace and take a breather whenever you feel in need of one.

Note: *If you are in the most advanced position for this exercise, you will not be able to lift your foot more than 1 inch, if that. If you are not yet strong enough for this, you may lean your torso over to the opposite side of your working leg to allow you to lift your leg higher – but make sure it is no more than 3 inches off the floor. Otherwise, because you may be tired, you might inadvertently turn your leg so that your knee faces the ceiling and begin working the front thigh muscles instead of the buttocks.*

ENTIRE BODY

Open and Close

For greater strength, energy and vitality.

> **Note:** *Do not attempt this exercise during the first three months of pregnancy.*

This exercise builds up tremendous strength throughout the entire body. The results are incredibly fast because you are using several sets of muscles – from your chest, upper back, arms and stomach (abdomen), to your legs and thighs. At the beginning, the more you do, the lower your legs will go. Expect this – don't think you're not doing the exercise correctly if it happens. Believe it or not, there are some people in their seventies who can do fifty Open and Closes effortlessly, without breathers, and their legs remain extremely high.

As with so much of Callanetics, this is an exercise that must be respected. Most people with back problems have found that Open and Close has helped their backs tremendously – because they knew their own limitations and did not force the exercise. This means they stopped when they felt the lower back was about to take over, and only did what they felt they could do at that particular time. Even though this is basically a leg exercise, it requires tremendous use of the stomach muscles as well. This is why, if your abdominals are not particularly strong, your lower back will inevitably take over – which is not what you want! Build yourself up slowly, and you'll soon find that another wonderful benefit of this exercise is that your entire body, especially your stomach muscles, also becomes stronger.

You should be totally relaxed when starting this exercise. If you have sciatica, keep your knees bent throughout.

Note: *For the barre in this exercise you can use any solid piece of furniture such as the back of a sofa or heavy chair. Some people use a sturdy chest of drawers with one drawer open. At first you will be hanging on for dear life, so before you begin make sure the object you will be holding on to is strong enough to support your weight. Use a mat or towel to cushion yourself if necessary.*

At first you will probably be opening and closing your legs across the floor, as Nina is demonstrating here. Height does not matter. Work at your own level. When your legs become stronger you will be able to lift your legs off the floor and your legs will feel like feathers.

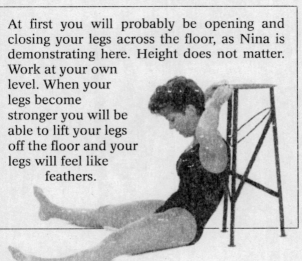

▶ Sit on the floor with your upper back against your barre or sturdy piece of furniture and hold on to the top of it as if there is a barre above your head. Bend your knees and take them in towards your chest. Point your toes. Scoot your buttocks forward 4 to 5 inches away from the furniture so that you are not sitting on your tailbone. This will take the pressure off your lower back. (When you scoot forward – shifting first one buttock and then the other – at the same time try to get the bottom of your pubic bone to round up and in towards your navel. It is similar doing the pelvic curl-up except that you do not have to tighten your buttocks.) Gently drop your chin. This will help to stretch your spine more.

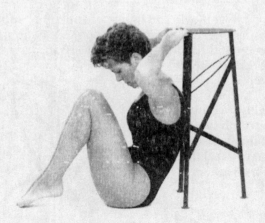

▶ Clasping your barre or furniture firmly with both hands, relax your shoulders and neck. Without locking your knees, slowly straighten your legs, raising them as high as you can without forcing, pointing your toes up towards the ceiling. You are sitting in a jackknife position. (If you are not able to lift your legs at first, straighten them out on the floor.) *In triple slow motion*, open your legs as wide as you can, and then close them.

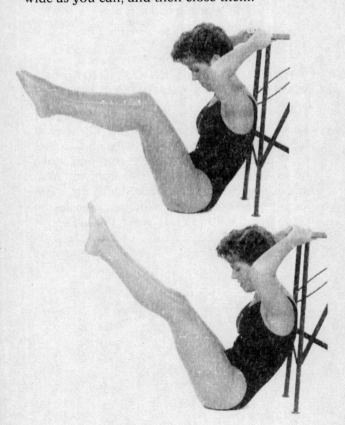

▶To come out of the exercise, gently bring your legs to the closed position and bend your knees, bringing your knees in close to your chest, then slowly lower your legs to the floor.

REPETITIONS

▶▶ Start with 2 sets of 5

▶▶ Work up to 4 sets of 5

IF YOU FEEL YOU ARE LOSING STRENGTH, OR YOUR LOWER BACK IS ABOUT TO TAKE OVER:

Lower your legs a few inches, or bend your knees as you open and close. Or take a breather. If you find that you're still feeling pressure on your lower back, stop and move on to the next exercise. Only return to Open and Close when you have built up more strength in your stomach and leg muscles by practising the other exercises in this series.

WHEN THIS EXERCISE BECOMES TOO EASY:

Move your buttocks closer to your barre or piece of furniture. It is much harder to raise your legs from this position – just try, and you'll understand. The higher you can raise your legs, the more challenging Open and Close becomes. It takes incredible strength to raise your legs high with ease. When you become very strong, instead of gripping the barre tightly you will need to use only one finger as a balance point and your legs will feel as light as feathers.

REMEMBER

- Before you begin, make sure the object you will be holding on to is sturdy enough to hold your weight. Until you become stronger you will be holding on for dear life.

- Take as many breathers as you wish. Do not overdo it. Gradually work up to 4 sets of 5, increasing slowly as your muscles tighten and strengthen.

- Relax your legs, especially the knees. Eventually your legs will feel as light as feathers.

continued ...

- Although your toes are pointed, keep your feet relaxed.

- Never force your legs further apart than they can comfortably go.

- Keep your chin down.

- Don't forget, Open and Close must be treated with the respect it deserves!

STRETCHING

The Sitting Hamstring Stretch

> *This exercise:*
>
> - stretches the neck, spine, the area between the shoulder blades, the inner thighs, and the backs of the legs, especially the hamstrings
> - strengthens the pectoral muscles

Note: *If you have sciatica, always keep your knees bent during this exercise.*

▶ Sit up on the floor with your shoulders erect, legs together and toes pointed but relaxed. Rest your hands on the front of your thighs and aim your elbows out to the sides to stretch the area between your shoulder blades. Stretch your torso up. Now, *very gently*, round your head and shoulders – like a cat stretching – aiming your nose and shoulders towards the top of your legs. Then,

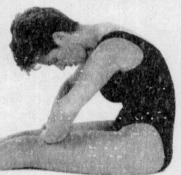

walking your hands forward on your legs, keep curling your upper torso until your head and shoulders are rounded as much as possible, without forcing. You will eventually be aiming to rest your head on your legs. Totally relax your body, letting it melt into the floor. Feel the beautiful stretch in your lower back and hamstrings. Now, *gently* pulse your upper torso up and down, no more than 1/4 to 1/2 inch, keeping your elbows relaxed and out to the sides.

▶ To come out of the stretch, slowly walk your hands back up your legs and gently round your upper torso up, one vertebra at a time, until you are sitting erect. Gently bring your head up last of all.

REPETITIONS
▶▶ 50 pulses

IF YOU'RE NOT VERY STRETCHED AND THIS EXERCISE IS TOO DIFFICULT, OR IF YOU FEEL PRESSURE IN YOUR LOWER BACK:

Do not take your torso over so far and keep your knees bent if you need to.

Do not worry if you can not straighten your legs completely at first. Just keep them bent as Nina's are here. As you become more stretched, you will be able to straighten your legs with ease.

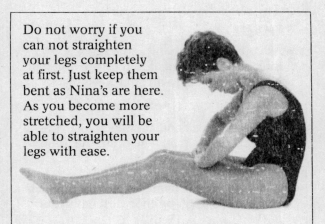

FOR MORE OF A STRETCH:

Walk your hands further down your legs, and round your upper torso over even more so that your head is resting on your legs. You can place your hands on the floor to the sides of you. For even more of a stretch in this position, especially for your calves, you can also flex your feet. This is such a relaxing position that some people feel like taking a nap!

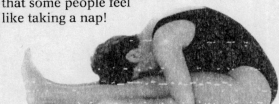

REMEMBER

- As you go down, your upper torso is rounded – not straight. Otherwise you will be putting pressure on your lower back.

- Relax your legs, especially your knees.

- Relax your neck and shoulders. Let your neck and entire body melt into the floor.

- Do not force your body down.

- As you do your tiny pulses, do not bounce or jerk, and don't pull forward with your neck.

- Feel the stretch in your lower back.

FRONT THIGHS

The Front-Thigh Stretch

For tight, slim beautiful thighs.

> **This exercise:**
>
> • stretches the front thighs, spine, neck and pectoral muscles
>
> • strengthens the buttocks, inner thighs and stomach

When I first started doing this stretch I felt incredible pressure on my knees. Since I have a history of knee problems I was terribly concerned that I might be aggravating my pre-existing condition. However, in the hope of avoiding knee surgery I was prepared to go through any amount of pain, believing that by going beyond the pain I could obtain relief. I therefore persevered with this exercise and found my knee problems improved tremendously, thereby saving me from the surgeon's knife. Many people have had similar experiences. If, in the beginning, you feel uncomfortable with this stretch and you choose to continue, you may find, as many others have, that the pressure on your knees eventually eases. However, you may choose to discontinue this stretch and return to it when your body becomes stronger from practising the other exercises in this series.

▶ Sit on your heels with your knees together and your feet relaxed. If necessary, use a pillow or towel to cushion your legs from knee to toe. Relax your shoulders. Now, lean back, placing your palms on the floor behind you, your fingers facing away from your body. Rest your weight on your heels, and relax your neck. Still sitting on your heels, tighten your buttocks and curl your pelvis up more than you think you can. Again, still sitting on your heels, curl your pelvis up even more.

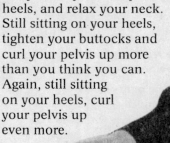

▶ Now, lift your buttocks up off your heels no more than 1 inch.

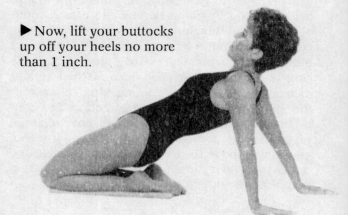

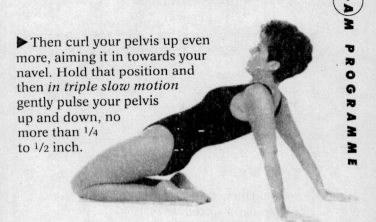

▶ Then curl your pelvis up even more, aiming it in towards your navel. Hold that position and then *in triple slow motion* gently pulse your pelvis up and down, no more than 1/4 to 1/2 inch.

▶ When you have finished your pulses, relax your buttocks and gently return to the starting position, sitting on your heels. Relax your entire body.

Note: *As you become stronger, you will be able to curl your pelvis up even more, while completely relaxing your entire body. In the photograph above, Nina's pelvis is curled up even higher, but, because the movement is so tiny and delicate, the naked eye can hardly see the difference between this and the preceding photograph. However, even though it is difficult to see, if you manage to curl your pelvis up this high you will certainly feel the difference!*

REPETITIONS

▶▶ Start with 10 pulses

▶▶ Work up to 20 pulses

IF THIS EXERCISE IS TOO DIFFICULT AT FIRST:

You can place your hands on the floor at each side of you. It may also be more comfortable in the beginning if you separate your knees a wee bit.

REMEMBER

- Keep your knees together and your shoulders relaxed.

- Keep your spine straight; do not arch your back.

- Do not tense your neck.

- Do not allow your head to drop back.

- Do not move your head up and down.

- Keep your arms straight but relaxed. Do not put too much pressure on your hands and do not lock your elbows.

- Do not tense your body.

- The more you can curl your pelvis up, aiming it in towards your navel, the more your front-thigh muscles will stretch to give them a long, sleek, tight look.

INNER THIGHS

The Inner-Thigh Squeeze

For lethal inner thighs!

> *This exercise:*
>
> - **tightens the inner thighs**
> - **stretches the spine**
> - **strengthens the stomach, buttocks, psoas, calves and feet**

For this exercise you will need a sturdy piece of furniture that you can squeeze with your legs, such as a stool, chair, the legs of a table or desk – even a filing cabinet. The width is not critical, as long as you are comfortable. Just make sure it's not fragile. You may be surprised at how strong your inner thighs will become as you do this powerful contraction.

▶ Facing the stool, chair, table or desk legs, sit on the floor, with your back straight, and let your hands rest on the floor by your sides. Bend your knees and place the arch of each foot around the outsides of the stool or table legs so that the toes of each foot are pointing towards each other. Gently round (curl) your upper torso so that you won't

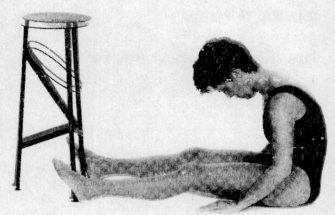

try to put pressure on your lower back. Take this opportunity to gently stretch the back of your neck by letting your head aim down towards your chest.

▶ Keeping your toes pointed and relaxed, squeeze your legs as much as you can, as if trying to bring the legs of your piece of furniture together. Squeeze for the count, if you can, then release. You will see better results if you squeeze continuously, instead of holding and relaxing. Your inner thighs are doing all the work.

> **HOLD FOR A COUNT OF...**
> ▶▶ Start with 75
> ▶▶ Work up to 100

WHEN THIS EXERCISE BECOMES TOO EASY:

Straighten your legs and raise your feet 1 to 4 inches off the floor. When your legs become stronger you can place the arches of your feet even higher up your piece of furniture.

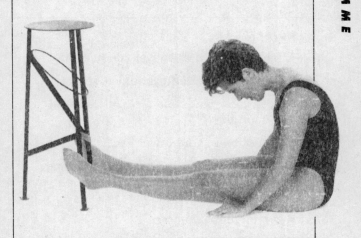

FOR EVEN MORE OF A CHALLENGE:

With your legs resting on the floor, place the inside of your heels on the outsides of the stool or table legs. Either point your toes away from the chair or table legs or point your toes upwards (whichever feels more comfortable) and squeeze with your heels.

Note: At first you will be tempted to arch your lower back to assist the inner-thigh muscles. Always keep your upper torso rounded. If you find your lower back is still assisting during the Inner-Thigh Squeeze, round your upper torso even more. You can also take breathers whenever you need to.

REMEMBER

- Take breathers whenever you need to.

- Keep your neck and shoulders relaxed.

- Keep your hands and arms relaxed and comfortable.

- Do not tense your lower back.

- Do not lean backward. Keep your upper torso rounded to take the pressure off your lower back.

- Do not tense your feet.

- Relax your body by letting it melt into the floor.

- When you are in one of the more advanced positions for this exercise, do not tense your legs or lock your knees.

Note: At first you will probably feel this exercise working in your calves and the insides of your knees. Just continue, and all of a sudden you will feel it in your inner thighs and realize just how much your inner thighs have been working all along.

Now that you have completed the **am programme**, I hope you are feeling a sense of wellbeing and calm exhilaration, and that you are ready to face the day with a smile. See you later for a wonderfully relaxing **pm** class.

Now it's time to shed the tensions of the day and achieve a beautiful tight body at the same time. Before you start on this **pm programme**, take a deep breath and give a lovely, powerful sigh. Now totally relax your body and mind, and leave the stresses of the day behind. Remember, Callanetics is meditation in motion. For the next twenty minutes, as you perform the exercises, concentrate fully on the wonderful benefits you are giving your body by doing these gentle, precise movements. By focusing your thoughts on each movement and allowing your body to be like a rag doll, you will leave the worries of the day behind as you create a stronger, healthier and more relaxed mind and body.

The pm Programme

WARM-UPS

The Swing

A gentle, sweeping movement.

> **This exercise:**
> - stretches the spine
> - loosens the knees

This is basically the same gentle, swinging stretch as Up and Down, except you will stay in a semi-crouching position.

▶ Stand with your feet a hip-width apart. Stretch both arms up towards the ceiling for a wonderful stretch. Bend your knees a little. Tighten your buttocks and curl your pelvis up. Now stretch your torso even more. Keep your knees relaxed and your feet flat on the floor. Now, gently bend your knees as much as you can and lower your upper body towards the floor, your arms reaching forward and aiming towards the floor.

WARM-UPS

▶ From this position, gently swing your arms backwards and then forward. Relax your entire body. You are a rag doll, sweeping your arms backward and forward as your knees gently move up and down.

▶ When you have finished your repetitions, tighten your buttocks and curl your pelvis up. Slowly return to your standing position, rounding up your torso vertebra by vertebra and bringing your head up last. Now stretch your arms up to the ceiling again for one last stretch.

REPETITIONS
▶▶ 5

REMEMBER

- Totally relax your knees.
- Keep your shoulders relaxed.
- Let go of your neck.
- Your entire body is relaxed, including your feet.

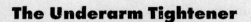

The Underarm Tightener

The only underarm exercise you'll ever need to do.

This exercise:

- tightens the underarms

- expands and stretches the chest

- stretches the spine and pectoral muscles

- loosens and relieves tension in the neck and the area between the shoulder blades

---

▶ Stand erect, with your feet a hip-width apart. Bend your knees a little. Take both arms up and out to the sides, keeping them perfectly straight and even with your shoulders. Slowly start rolling your hands forward, turning your wrists over so that your palms are face up, thumbs aiming towards the ceiling. Now, with your knees still bent slightly, tighten your buttocks and curl your pelvis up even more than you think you can, to protect your lower back. Make sure your spine is straight and your head is erect. Raise your shoulders to stretch your spine even more.

▶ Gently take your arms behind your back. Your shoulders will drop when your arms are taken to the back. Try to keep your hands as high as your shoulders and your arms straight. Without jerking, *slowly* move your arms 1/4 to 1/2 inch closer together and back in gentle, tiny pulsing movements, trying to get your thumbs to touch each other. After a few of these movements, gravity will start to pull your arms down and your head and shoulders forward. Be aware of this, and try to return them to the proper position. You may find it difficult to keep your elbows straight at first. Keep trying and eventually it will happen. Also, keep your wrists turned and your body erect.

REPETITIONS
▶▶ Start with 75 pulses
▶▶ Work up to 100 pulses

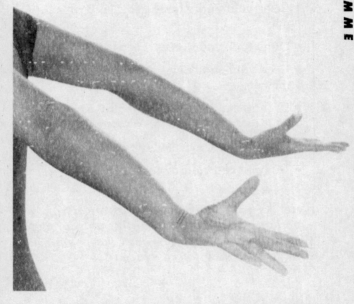

Note: See how much the wrists are turned. The more your wrists are turned over and your thumbs and fingers aimed towards the ceiling, and the higher and straighter you can hold your arms, the more you will be working your underarms and loosening the area between your shoulder blades.

PM PROGRAMME

REMEMBER

- Keep your pelvis curled up.

- Do not allow gravity to pull your arms down. Keep them as high as you can.

- Relax your entire body, especially your neck.

- Don't lock your knees; keep them relaxed.

- Keep your shoulders pulled back and relaxed.

- Do not lean your torso forward. Keep your torso stretched up towards the ceiling.

- Do not take your head forward.

- Do not bend your elbows.

Note: As your body becomes stronger you will experience no difficulty in curling up your pelvis. When this happens you may keep your legs straight with your knees relaxed.

The Standing Hamstring Stretch

This exercise:

- stretches the hamstring muscles, calves, lower back and the area between the shoulder blades

Note: *If you have mild sciatica, always keep your knees bent during this exercise. If you have more than mild sciatica, you can substitute the Lying-Down Hamstring Stretch on page 147.*

▶ Stand erect with feet a hip-width apart. Bend your knees and, *without forcing*, very slowly round your torso over in front as much as you can *without forcing*, trying to aim your head down towards your knees. Keep your body relaxed and your head tucked under. Now, gently grasp the insides of each ankle with both hands and aim your elbows out to the sides to stretch the area between your shoulder blades. *In triple slow motion*, pulse your torso ¼ to ½ inch, trying to ease your head between your legs, without forcing. Do not bounce. Relax your shoulders and neck and let your body melt into the floor.

►When you have completed your repetitions, *gently* move your torso over to your right side. Clasp your right ankle with both hands, your right hand on the inside of the ankle and your left hand on the outside. Your elbows are aimed out to the sides and your knees are still bent. Try to ease your head in between your right arm and right leg as far as it will go without forcing. In triple slow motion, pulse your torso no more than ¼ to ½ inch. Relax even more.

►Keeping your knees relaxed, *gently* move your torso over to your left side, clasping your left ankle with both hands, your left hand on the inside of the ankle, and your right hand on the outside. Keep your elbows bent and aimed out to the sides. Try to ease your head between your left arm and left leg and gently pulse your torso ¼ to ½ inch.

▶To come out of this stretch, *in triple slow motion*, gently move your torso back to the centre and, with your legs relaxed, let your body and arms hang loosely, like a rag doll. Then bend your knees as much as you possibly can, lowering your buttocks towards the floor so you are in a crouching position. Now, tighten your buttocks, curl your pelvis up and, letting your arms hang loosely in front, *slowly* round your torso up, vertebra by vertebra, to return to your original standing position, Gently bring your head up last of all.

REPETITIONS
in each position
▶▶ **20 pulses to the centre**
▶▶ **20 pulses to the right**
▶▶ **20 pulses to the left**

Note: At first, some people will not be able to reach over as far as Nina demonstrates here. Just work at your own pace and in no time at all your muscles will have much more elasticity.

FOR EVEN MORE OF A STRETCH:

Move your feet closer together. (You must have good balance for this position.)

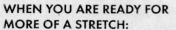

WHEN YOU ARE READY FOR MORE OF A STRETCH:

Keep your legs straight throughout the exercise, but do not lock your knees. The more stretched you are, the more you will be able to straighten your legs, keeping the knees relaxed. Notice how rounded Nina's torso is.

Note: Take advantage of this time to relax your neck. It should feel as if it is melting into the floor.

REMEMBER

- Do not force.

- Do not tense or lock the knees.

- Keep your entire back relaxed.

- Keep your pulses fluid and small. *Never jerk or bounce.*

- Relax your neck.

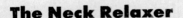
The Neck Relaxer

A way to unlock tension.

> **This exercise:**
> - loosens the neck and shoulders
> - stretches the spine
> - increases joint flexibility
> - releases tension in the neck and the area between the shoulder blades

▶ Stand erect, feet a hip-width apart, knees relaxed. Relax your entire body, letting your shoulders melt into the floor. Be careful not to arch your lower back or stick out your stomach. If you have a tendency to do this, tighten your buttocks and curl your pelvis up more than you think you can. Now, *in triple slow motion*, take your head down to rest your chin on your chest.

113

▶Still slowly, move your chin over to your right shoulder as far as you can. Then aim your chin up towards the ceiling as high as you can, stretching the back of your neck up. Delicately bring your chin back down to your chest.

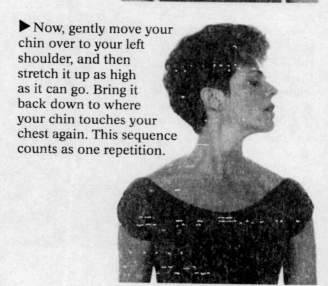

▶Now, gently move your chin over to your left shoulder, and then stretch it up as high as it can go. Bring it back down to where your chin touches your chest again. This sequence counts as one repetition.

> **REPETITIONS**
> to each side
> 3

REMEMBER

- Do not hunch or tense your shoulders; keep them relaxed. Imagine you are letting them drip into the floor.

- Do not move your shoulders when you are moving your head either to your right or left side.

- Do not make any harsh or sudden movements.

- Do not tense your jaw.

- Keep your knees relaxed; don't lock them.

- Do not stick out your stomach or arch your lower back.

Note: *Remember to do this exercise* in triple slow motion, *with your shoulders melting into the floor and your body like a rag doll.*

STOMACH

The Bent-Knee Reach

You'll never do another sit-up.

For the benefits of this and the next exercise, see page 50.

▶Lie on the floor, knees bent, feet a hip-width apart and flat on the floor. Your arms are by your sides. Relax your shoulders. *With your head still on the floor*, grasp your inner thighs with all your might. Take your elbows out to the sides as much as you can, and them aim them up towards the ceiling to stretch your upper-back muscles.

▶Letting the lower part of your back be relaxed and melting into the floor, slowly round your head and shoulders off the floor, aiming your nose and shoulders in towards your chest. At the same time, bring your elbows out and up towards the ceiling even more, all the while grasping your inner thighs for dear life.

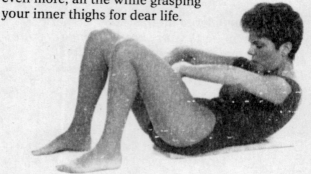

▶ When your head and shoulders are rounded as much as possible, take your hands off your thighs and gently lower your arms to the sides of your legs, aiming them straight to the front of you, palms down, about 6 to 12 inches off the floor. Now, *in triple slow motion*, gently pulse your upper torso forward and back no more than 1/4 to 1/2 inch. Totally relax your buttocks and your middle- and lower back by letting them melt into the floor. Try to keep your head and shoulders rounded and aimed in towards your chest as much as you can.

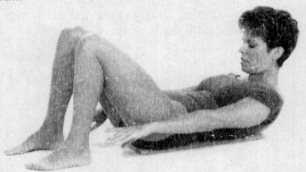

▶ To come out of this exercise, *in triple slow motion* lower your head and shoulders back to the floor, rolling down one vertebra at a time.

REPETITIONS
▶▶ Start with 75 pulses
▶▶ Work up to 100 pulses

117

IF YOU NEED TO TAKE A BREATHER:

Without returning to the floor, grasp your inner thighs with your hands, as in the starting position, and hold your rounded position while you rest. Then, before releasing your hands to continue the exercise, take your elbows out and then up, and then round your head and shoulders even more, aiming your nose and shoulders in towards your chest. Or, you may roll down vertebra by vertebra to rest on the floor – but remember, if you choose this option you must start at Step 1 again when continuing with the exercise.

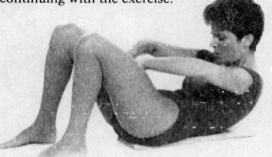

IF YOU FEEL DISCOMFORT IN YOUR NECK THE FIRST FEW TIMES:

Grasp your hands behind your head, letting your head rest in the palms of your hands and keeping your elbows out to the sides.

IF YOU FEEL A STRAIN IN YOUR LOWER BACK:

This is usually because your are tensing your lower-back muscles instead of letting your lower back be relaxed by melting it into the floor.

Note: Be sure to maintain that fabulous round! If your shoulders fall back a bit at first, don't worry. In the beginning, most people's stomach muscles are not yet strong enough to hold the position. When your muscles become stronger, do not allow your shoulders to drop back.

IF YOU FEEL THERE IS A STRAIN ON YOUR LOWER BACK OR THAT YOUR ENTIRE BODY IS MOVING BACK AND FORTH ON THE FLOOR:

Lift your feet 1 to 2 inches up off the floor, or move your feet very slightly away from your body; or take your shoulders down to the floor 1/2 inch at a time until you feel no strain on your back. Moving back and forth or in a jerking motion is your signal that your back muscles are trying to come to assist your stomach muscles.

REMEMBER

- Do not tense your stomach muscles. This puts pressure on your lower back. Your stomach muscles will be doing enough work.

- Do not tense your body. Just relax and let your lower back melt into the floor.

- Try not to let your shoulders sink back down to the floor. Keep them rounded off the floor as much as possible.

- Do not move just your arms or your shoulders or neck when pulsing. They all move together with your upper torso as a unit.

- Do not tense your buttocks. They should not move at all. Relaxing them will ensure your lower back does not try to take over.

- Keep your legs and neck relaxed.

- Never aim your face towards the ceiling. Always aim your nose and shoulders in towards your rib cage.

- Do not jerk or bounce.

- Take breathers whenever you need to.

Remember, if you should come up off the floor after any of these exercises, re-read the instructions on pages 48–49 on how to get up properly without putting pressure on your back.

The Double-Leg Raise

▶ Lying on the floor with your knees bent and feet a hip-width apart, bend one knee at a time in towards your chest, then extend each leg in turn straight up towards the ceiling, with toes pointed and relaxed. (Don't worry if you can't straighten your legs completely at first.)

▶ Grasp your outer thighs with both hands and take your elbows out to the sides and then up as high as you can. Gently round your head and shoulders off the floor, aiming your nose and shoulders in towards your chest, and take your elbows out and up even more.

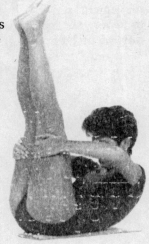

▶ When you feel you can't round any further, take your hands off your thighs and place them by your sides, extending them straight out in front, palms down, 6 inches to 1 foot off the floor. *In triple slow motion*, gently pulse your torso forward and back, no more than 1/4 to 1/2 inch.

▶ When you feel comfortable with this movement, start to lower your legs only 1/2 inch at a time.

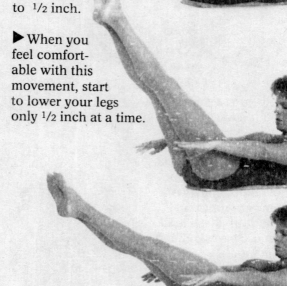

The lower your legs go down to the floor, the more your stomach muscles work. But only lower them as far as you can without feeling any strain in your lower back. If your lower back is starting to arch, again, this is your signal that your stomach muscles are not yet strong enough to work at this level. Slowly raise your legs back up in ½-inch segments until you feel absolutely no discomfort in your lower back, or your lower back does not arch, and then continue the exercise at that level.

▶ To come out of this exercise, *in triple slow motion* gently bend first your right knee and then your left knee in towards your chest, and lower your feet to the floor, one at a time. Then gently lower your head and shoulders back to the floor, rolling down vertebra by vertebra.

REPETITIONS

▶▶ Start with 75 pulses

▶▶ Work up to 100 pulses

IF YOU NEED TO TAKE A BREATHER:

Grasp your outer thighs with both hands and hold your rounded position, with your elbows still aimed out to the sides, and breathe deeply and naturally. Before letting go to continue the count, round your head and shoulders even more and bring your elbows up and out more than you think you can.

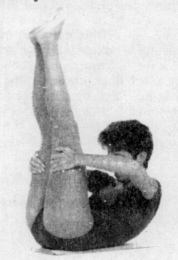

IF THIS EXERCISE IS TOO DIFFICULT AT FIRST:

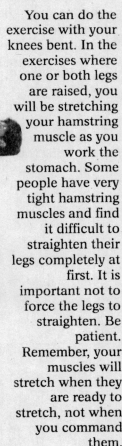

You can do the exercise with your knees bent. In the exercises where one or both legs are raised, you will be stretching your hamstring muscle as you work the stomach. Some people have very tight hamstring muscles and find it difficult to straighten their legs completely at first. It is important not to force the legs to straighten. Be patient. Remember, your muscles will stretch when they are ready to stretch, not when you command them.

FOR MORE OF A CHALLENGE:

When your muscles become extremely strong you will eventually be able to take your legs to where they are 2 to 4 inches off the floor. There should be no strain on your body at all. Your lower back should always be on the floor, not arched. It takes incredible strength to lower your legs and still have your body feeling like a rag doll melting into the floor. Do not force. If you need to take a breather, you will have to gently bring your legs back up to a comfortable position so that you can easily hold on to your outer thighs.

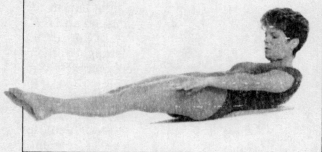

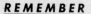

REMEMBER

- Your elbows must be up and out as far as they can possibly go for the starting position.

- Keep your head and shoulders rounded off the floor, aiming your nose and shoulders in towards your chest.

- Keep your entire body relaxed. Especially relax your legs and neck. Your legs should feel like feathers.

- Do not tense your buttocks or stomach muscles.

- Do not let your lower back arch or come up off the floor. This is your signal that your stomach muscles are not quite strong enough to maintain that position. If so, raise your legs in $1/2$-inch segments until you have reached a comfortable position. Concentrate on letting your lower back melt into the floor.

INNER THIGHS

The Inner-Thigh Stretch

> *This exercise:*
>
> • stretches the inner thighs, spine, neck, underarms and legs

Note: *Keep your torso relaxed during this exercise. Never force your legs further apart than they can go. If you have a tendency to sciatic pain, always keep your knees bent during this exercise. This will help relieve the pressure. If that is not helpful, discontinue this stretch until you are free from pain.*

▶ Sitting on the floor, spread your legs as far apart as they can go without forcing. Place your palms on the floor either in front or to the back of you.

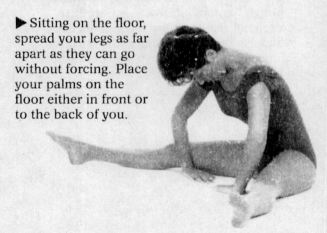

128

Gently push your pubic bone into the floor, and then scoot it forward a wee bit for a better stretch. Stretch your torso up, place your hands on your upper thighs or on the floor in front of you. Take your elbows out to the sides, and round your upper back so that you are not putting pressure on your lower back. Relax your shoulders and your neck. Now, stretch your shoulders up and, *in triple slow motion*, round your upper back forward and down – like a cat stretching – until your head and shoulders are down towards the floor as far as they can go without straining. Relax your body, and feel the stretch in your lower back and inner thighs. Stretch only as far as you are comfortable. Now, gently pulse your torso $1/4$ to $1/2$ inch, up and down.

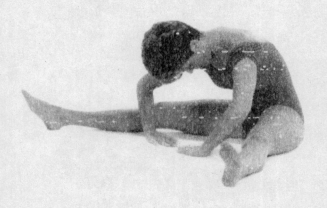

INNER THIGHS

▶When you have completed your repetitions, slowly walk your hands across the floor to the right and move your torso over to your right leg. Gently criss-cross your hands on your leg (wherever it is comfortable for you, but *not* on your knee) and aim your elbows out to the sides. In an almost imperceptible motion, pulse your torso towards your feet, 1/4 to 1/2 inch, aiming your head down towards your leg to stretch your neck. Eventually you will be aiming to rest your head on your legs.

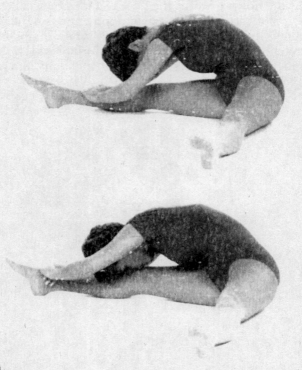

▶Next you will be going over to the left. Again, slowly walk your hands across the floor, moving your torso over to your left leg. Gently criss-cross your hands on your leg, aiming your elbows out, and repeat your tiny pulsing movements. Relax your neck, shoulders, feet – relax your entire body, letting it melt into the floor.

▶To come out of this stretch, gently walk your hands back to the centre and then walk them back up, slowly rounding up your torso, vertebra by vertebra, to return to your original sitting position.

REPETITIONS
in each position

▶▶ 50 pulses to the centre

▶▶ 50 pulses to the right

▶▶ 50 pulses to the left

TO GET A BETTER STRETCH IN YOUR WAIST:

As you do your tiny pulses to the right or to the left, try to aim the opposite elbow towards your foot (your left elbow to your right foot, or your right elbow to your left foot).

IF THIS EXERCISE IS TOO DIFFICULT AT FIRST:

Bend your knees as much as you have to and place your hands on your upper thighs, aiming your elbows out to the sides. Do your delicate pulses from this position. As you become more stretched you will be able to straighten your legs and move your torso closer towards the floor. Always relax.

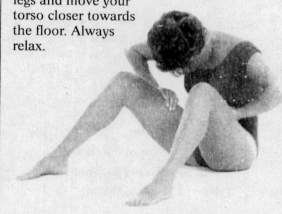

WHEN THIS EXERCISE BECOMES TOO EASY:

Stretch your legs further apart and keep them flat on the floor. When you are more stretched you will be able to touch the floor with either your forehead, your nose or your upper torso, but never force your body down or stretch more than is comfortable. Your muscles will stretch in their own time. When you are eventually able to rest your body on the floor, take advantage of this time to let your body completely relax and melt into the floor.

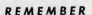

REMEMBER

- Do not force or bounce your body down.
- Do not pull forward with your neck.
- Relax your toes and your legs.
- Do not lock your knees.
- Relax your entire body, especially your neck and upper back.

continued ...

- Never force your legs further apart than they can comfortably go.
- Keep your elbows out and away from your body to stretch the area between your shoulder blades.

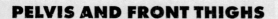
PELVIS AND FRONT THIGHS

The Pelvic Rotation

Beautiful, flowing, seductive.

This exercise:

- strengthens the buttocks, thighs, inner thighs, lower back, stomach, feet, and pelvic muscles
- stretches the arms and spine
- loosens the pelvic area

You may find this exercise difficult at first because it draws strength from your entire body. However, once you have mastered this rotation, it will give you incredible control of your pelvic area. Loosening the pelvic area is important. The legs and torso are influenced by it tremendously, and if this area is tight you won't have the flexibility that everyone is entitled to. This exercise can help you regain the wonderful, youthful suppleness and sense of freedom you had as a child.

At first, some people experience some discomfort in their knees. If this happens, continue to do the exercise very gently but with your knees slightly apart. Soon the discomfort should subside, unless you have a medical problem.

135

If you have knee problems and you find this too uncomfortable, you can do the Pelvic Rotation in a standing position, with your knees bent, feet a hip-width apart and facing forward. You will not see results as quickly, but your safety is far more important! Most people with knee problems have experienced wonderful results from this exercise and the next one.

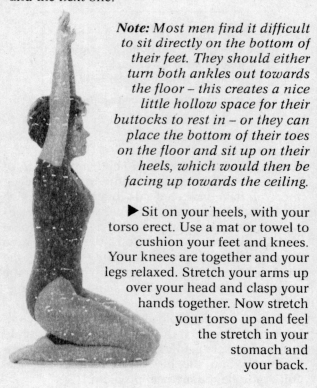

Note: *Most men find it difficult to sit directly on the bottom of their feet. They should either turn both ankles out towards the floor – this creates a nice little hollow space for their buttocks to rest in – or they can place the bottom of their toes on the floor and sit up on their heels, which would then be facing up towards the ceiling.*

▶ Sit on your heels, with your torso erect. Use a mat or towel to cushion your feet and knees. Your knees are together and your legs relaxed. Stretch your arms up over your head and clasp your hands together. Now stretch your torso up and feel the stretch in your stomach and your back.

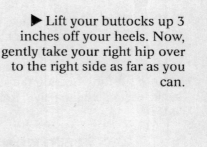

▶ Lift your buttocks up 3 inches off your heels. Now, gently take your right hip over to the right side as far as you can.

▶ Tighten your buttocks and curl your pelvis up, and at the same time roll your pelvis forward, to the front, aiming it up and in towards your navel. Now, move your left hip over to the left side as far as you can. Then move your buttocks to the back, completing a circle. One complete circle counts as one repetition.

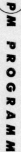
▶ Working at your own pace, complete the repetitions to this side, moving *in triple slow motion* as you circle to the right, front, left and back. Take a breather for a few seconds, then lift yourself back up into position, feeling the stretch in your lower back, and repeat the Pelvic Rotation starting to the left.

REPETITIONS
in each direction
▶▶ Start off with 3
▶▶ Work up to 5

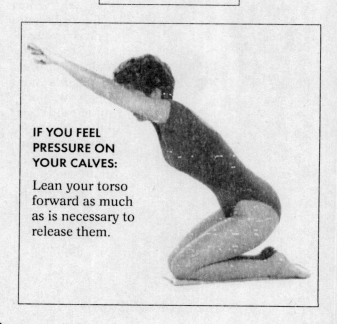

IF YOU FEEL PRESSURE ON YOUR CALVES:

Lean your torso forward as much as is necessary to release them.

Note: *If you find it difficult to maintain the position with your buttocks lifted 3 inches off your heels, you can lift your buttocks up further until you are comfortable.*

REMEMBER

- Keep your entire body relaxed.

- The more you can curl your pelvis up and in towards your navel when rolling your pelvis forward, the more effective this exercise.

- The entire movement should be one smooth, flowing circle – hip – pelvis – hip – behind. Only your pelvis moves.

- Take breathers whenever you need to.

- Do not arch your back or stick out your stomach.

The Pelvic Scoop

Graceful, gentle, sensuous.

> *This exercise:*
> - strengthens the leg muscles, especially the front- and inner thigh muscles, the stomach, buttocks, and calves
> - stretches the spine

▶ Kneel on a mat, knees together, with your feet outstretched behind you and your legs relaxed. Keep your arms and shoulders relaxed and your spine straight.

Lift your arms up and over your head, stretching as high as possible, and clasp your hands together. Feel the stretch in your lower back. Lower your arms about a foot in front of you, and round your upper torso forward as if you were diving into a pool.

▶ Now, keeping your spine straight, aim your buttocks towards the back, at the same time *aiming* them down towards your heels and still feeling the stretch in your spine. Do not simply sit down on your heels and do *not* arch your back.

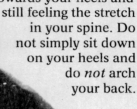

▶ When you have stretched your buttocks to the point where they are delicately brushing your heels, gently tighten your buttocks, and then curl your pelvis up even more than you think you can, in a slow, scooping motion. Hold for a split second and, if you can, raise your arms back up until your hands are above your head in the starting position. Then keep curling your pelvis up, and use the strength of your thighs to lift your body back up to the original kneeling position. When your pelvis is curled up, your buttocks will be closer to your heels.

REPETITIONS
▶▶ Work up to 5

Note: *The stronger you are, the more you will be able to take your arms towards the back when you are scooping back up in triple slow motion. Also, the more your can take your arms and torso back when you are returning to the original kneeling position with your curl-up, the faster your thigh muscles will strengthen. This is, however, quite a challenge. And the higher you can curl your pelvis, the more you will be strengthening your inner thighs.*

IF YOU FEEL A STRAIN OR A PULL IN YOUR CALVES WHEN YOU ARE RETURNING TO THE ORIGINAL KNEELING POSITION:

Take your arms and torso forward until almost parallel to the floor. After doing the scoop regularly you will soon be able to relax your calves and do the exercise in the usual way without thinking about it.

FOR MORE OF A CHALLENGE:

Push your knees together when you are returning to the original kneeling position.

REMEMBER

- Keep your entire body relaxed.
- Keep your arms and shoulders relaxed.
- Keep your pelvis curled up when you are returning to your original kneeling position.
- Do not arch your back when aiming your buttocks to the back and down towards your heels.
- Do not strain your calves. Take your arms and torso forward if necessary to release them.
- Keep your buttocks tightened when you are returning to your original kneeling position.
- Do not keep going relentlessly. If you find yourself needing a breather, take one. Relax your body and breathe naturally, then resume the original position and continue.

The Front-Thigh Stretch

For sleeker, tighter, longer-looking thighs.

▶ Sit on your heels, with your knees together and feet relaxed. Relax your shoulders. Lean back, resting your weight on your heels and placing your palms on the floor behind you, with fingers facing away from your body. Relax your neck. Still sitting on your heels, tighten your buttocks and curl your pelvis up, aiming it in towards your navel, then curl it up even more.

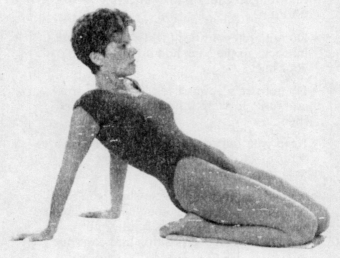

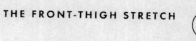

▶ Now, lift your buttocks up off your heels no more than 1 inch. Then curl your pelvis up even higher. *In triple slow motion*, gently pulse your pelvis up and down, still aiming it in towards your navel, no more than 1/4 to 1/2 inch.

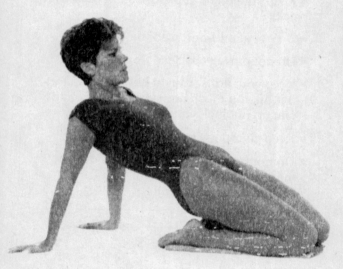

▶ When you have completed your pulses, relax your buttocks and slowly return to the starting position, sitting on your heels. Relax your entire body.

> **REPETITIONS**
> ▶▶ 10 pulses

REMEMBER

- Keep your knees together and your shoulders relaxed.

- Keep your spine straight; do not arch your back.

- Do not allow your head to drop back.

- Do not move your head up and down.

- Keep your arms straight but relaxed. Do not put too much pressure on your hands and do not lock your elbows.

- Keep your body relaxed; don't tense it.

- Do not forget to curl your pelvis up. The more you do this, the more your front thigh muscles will stretch.

STRETCHING

The Lying-Down Hamstring Stretch

This exercise:

- stretches the inner thighs, the backs of the legs (especially the hamstrings), the neck, spine, and the area between the shoulder blades

- strengthens the pectoral muscles

Note: If you have sciatica, always keep your knees bent during this exercise.

▶ Lie on your back, with your knees bent and feet a hip-width apart. Try to flatten the back of your neck on the floor. Bend your right knee up in towards

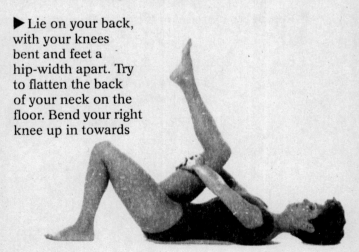

147

your chest, and then slowly straighten the leg as much as you can, aiming it upwards, *without forcing*. Do not worry if you are not able to straighten the leg at first – this is natural. Clasp your hands behind your right thigh, just below the knee. Take your elbows out and up to stretch the area between your shoulder blades and gently bring your leg as close to your body as you can. *In triple slow motion*, move your right leg towards you and back, pulsing for 1/4 to 1/2 inch. Always keep your elbows out, but make sure they are relaxed.

▶ To protect your back when coming out of this stretch or when switching sides to work the other leg, release your arms and, *in triple slow motion*, bring your right knee in towards your chest and place your foot flat on the floor.

▶ Repeat the exercise on the opposite side.

> **REPETITIONS**
> to each side
> ▶▶ 50

IF THIS EXERCISE IS TOO DIFFICULT AT FIRST:

Just hold your leg in the raised position for a count of 50, without pulsing.

WHEN THIS EXERCISE BECOMES TOO EASY AND YOU ARE READY FOR MORE OF A STRETCH:

Straighten your right leg as much as you can, without forcing, and gently ease your left leg down until it rests, fully extended, on the floor. Don't lock the knees. The more stretched you become, the lower your right leg will go down towards your head. To come out of this stretch and to switch sides, slowly bend your right knee into your chest and, with the knee bent, place your right foot flat on the floor. Bend your left knee in towards your chest and slowly straighten it up towards the ceiling as much as you can. Then gently slide your right leg down until it rests, fully extended, on the floor.

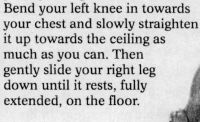

FOR EVEN MORE OF A STRETCH:

Hold your right leg at the ankle and take your leg down further towards the floor to the back of you. To take advantage of stretching the calf muscle, flex your right foot towards you. Do not point it up towards the ceiling.

REMEMBER

- Do not force your leg up higher than it can comfortably go.

- Do not lock your knees.

- Keep your resting leg on the floor. In the more advanced position, keep it as straight as possible but with the knee relaxed.

- Keep the foot of your raised leg pointed but relaxed.

continued ...

- Do not tighten your grasp on your thigh or ankle.

- Keep your elbows out and up.

- Keep your neck and shoulders very relaxed. Take advantage of this time to relax your entire body.

The Spine Stretch

Take advantage of this wonderful stretch as much as you can.

> *This exercise:*
>
> • stretches the entire back, spine, the area between the shoulder blades, the pectorals, buttocks, hips, and outer thighs

▶ Lying on the floor, with knees bent and feet flat on the floor, extend your arms out at shoulder level, elbows bent up at right angles, so that the backs of your hands rest on the floor. Your wrists might not touch the floor, but your elbows should always remain on the floor. Gently bring your right knee up towards your chest. Let your left leg gently ease down so that it is fully extended and resting on the floor.

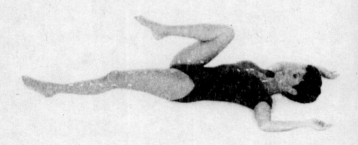

▶ Keeping both elbows on the floor, take your bent right knee over to your left side, away from your body as much as you can. *In triple slow motion*, pulse your left knee and leg up and down, 1/4 to 1/2 inch.

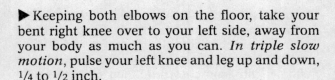

▶ When you have become more stretched, gravity will bring your right foot and then your right knee nearer to the ground, and eventually your foot and then your knee will be resting on the floor.

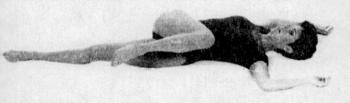

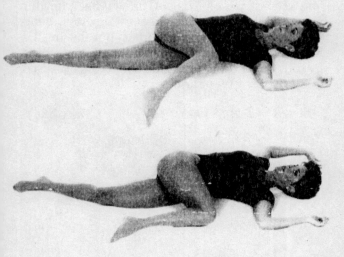

▶ To go over to the other side, in *triple slow motion*, keeping your right knee bent, bring it back to your chest and then place your right foot on the floor, with your knee still bent. Bend your left knee into your chest, and then slide your right foot down to the floor. This is all done in one smooth, continuous motion.

▶ Repeat this stretch on the opposite side.

> **REPETITIONS**
> to each side
> ▶▶ Work up to 50 pulses

To come out of this stretch, *in triple slow motion* and keeping your knee bent, bring it back to your chest, and then place your foot on the floor. Bend your other knee, and place that foot flat on the floor. Then ease yourself up to a standing position by rolling over on to your side and easing yourself up gently using your arms.

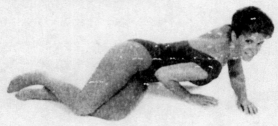

FOR MORE OF A STRETCH:

When you are stretched enough to allow your right foot and knee to rest on the floor, try to gently move your right knee up towards your left elbow.

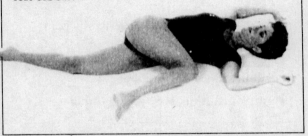

FOR EVEN MORE OF A STRETCH:

Ease your straight leg to the back of you.

Note: You will have to be very stretched to be able to get your right knee to touch the floor, without lifting your right elbow. Do not force the knee down. If you are not yet ready for such a stretch, it is more beneficial to keep your elbow on the floor and the knee in the air than to allow the elbow to come off the floor (as it will tend to do) in order to get your knee to touch the floor.

155

REMEMBER

- Do not force your bent leg down to the floor.

- Do not lift your shoulders or elbows off the floor.

- Relax your entire body, especially your neck.

- Do not force anything. Remember, gravity is doing the work, not you.

- Think beautiful, soft, gentle thoughts!

Doesn't that feel good! Now you have completed the **pm programme** you are ready for a relaxing evening, free from all the stresses of the day. Have a peaceful night's sleep, and I'll see you in the morning for **am Callanetics**.

ABOUT THE AUTHOR

Callan Pinckney was raised in Savannah, Georgia. She trained in classical ballet for twelve years and has studied other forms of dance, movement and exercise. She had to restore her own body to health when, after an eleven-year backpacking odyssey around the world, the rigours of travel, combined with a congenital back defect, led to physical collapse. On her return to the U.S. she experimented with various exercise techniques, using her early ballet training to develop the programme which finally solved her physical problems. Callan has taught her revolutionary exercise programme for over fifteen years and has had many famous and distinguished clients worldwide, all of whom testify that Callanetics is a unique, safe exercise system for transforming bodyshape.